Intermittent Fasting for Ageless Women Over 50 & 60

13 Secrets to Beat Menopause & Radiate Confidence Even in Your 50s and Beyond

Detox Your Body With 100+ Easy-To-Make Recipes & Boost Your Energy

Olivia Craig

Legal & Disclaimer

The information contained in this book and its contents is not designed to replace or take the place of any form of medical or professional advice and is not meant to replace the need for independent medical, financial, legal, or other professional advice or services, as may be required. The content and information in this book have been provided for educational and entertainment purposes only.

The content and information in this book have been compiled from reliable sources, and it is accurate to the best of the Author's knowledge, information, and belief. However, the Author cannot guarantee its accuracy and validity and cannot be held liable for errors and omissions. Further, changes are periodically made to this book as and when needed. Where appropriate and necessary, you must consult a professional (including but not limited to your doctor, attorney, financial advisor, or other professional advisor) before using any of the suggested remedies, techniques, or information in this book. Upon using the contents and information contained in this book, you agree to hold harmless the Author from and against any damages, costs, and expenses, including any legal fees potentially resulting from the application of any of the information provided by this book. This disclaimer applies to any loss, damages, or injury caused by the use and application, whether directly or indirectly, of any advice or information presented, whether for breach of contract, tort, negligence, personal injury, criminal intent, or under any other cause of action.

You agree to accept all risks of using the information presented in this book.

You agree that by continuing to read this book, where appropriate and necessary, you shall consult a professional (including but not limited to your doctor, attorney, financial advisor, or such other advisor as needed) before using any of the suggested remedies, techniques, or information in this book.

About the Author

Olivia Craig is a 54-year-old renowned health and wellness expert specializing in nutrition and fitness for women.

Due to long hours at a desk and a love for indulgent foods, Oliva's life turned sedentary. Over time, her health started deteriorating, and she decided to fight back. She embraced a new lifestyle filled with a healthy diet and daily exercise.

She reclaimed her life with **perseverance and hard work** and has dedicated her career to helping women embrace a healthy and vibrant lifestyle. Her passion for weight management and overall well-being has led her to write many research papers and books on this niche.

Olivia's expertise and research-based approach provide practical guidance, **ensuring her readers achieve sustainable results**.

Through her writing, she empowers women to **take charge of their health, harness their inner strength, and thrive in their golden years**.

When she's not writing, you can find Emily exploring nature trails, experimenting with new recipes in the kitchen, or sharing her knowledge through workshops and seminars.

Get Your Copy of Her Latest Writing Today and Bring A Positive Change In Your Life.

Table of Contents

Introduction

Reading this book and embarking on an active and healthy lifestyle is one of your best choices! Here, you will find what it means to stay agile, healthy, and fabulous as you fast.

Aging is an extraordinary process where you become the person you always should have been – David Bowie.

Aging is inevitable, but it doesn't mean you let go of your health and vitality. You can slow down the aging clock and enjoy life fully with the right strategies.

I do not have a PhD in nutrition, but I have collected ample knowledge about aging women and their body changes. In all these studies and research, I have found some common practices that positively affect an aging body.

Intermittent fasting is one such strategy that has numerous health benefits.

I wrote this book specifically for women over 50 and 60 looking to make the right health choices and want to gain knowledge regarding intermittent fasting before diving into it.

Like you, I have been living in a fool's paradise and thought skipping meals and only eating at a specific time would take me nowhere.

Fasting seemed difficult and drastic, and I thought, like many other diets – it was destined to fail. But as I looked deeper and experienced it myself, I can safely say that if it can do wonders for me, it can surely do it for you!

I have interviewed many medical experts and have plowed through hundreds of books to understand and pen how aging and fasting can go side by side.

You might have noticed the body changes as you age and that you can no longer rely on the same old diet and exercise routine that worked well in your younger days.

That's where intermittent fasting comes in - *it is a flexible and workable way of eating that helps improve your health markers, lose weight, and even extend your lifespan.*

But, like other things in life – it comes with a catch. You need to understand that intermittent fasting is not a universal approach. Women over 50 and 60 experience hormonal changes in their bodies, and that makes it somewhat challenging to stick to a single diet.

So, I have tailored the book by considering all these pointers. You will find different sections addressing women's problems in their 50s and 60s.

Furthermore, you will learn the following:

- Basics Of Intermittent Fasting And Is It Even Workable For You
- Benefits That Women Over 50 And 60 Can Expect From Intermittent Fasting
- Common Mistakes Women Do When They Start Fasting
- Best Practices For Fasting Comfortably And Safely
- Role Of Exercise, Sleep Cycle, And Nutrition In Supporting The Fast
- 100+ Delicious And Nutritious Recipes To Help You Plan Your Meals

But wait, this book is not just about intermittent fasting; this is an empowering guide that can help you make the best version of yourself.

From stress management to sleep, we've covered all the tips and tricks to help you feel good from the inside out.

And let's not forget about the bonus tools - we've included a list of the best mobile applications packed with food journals, progress trackers, and checklists to keep you accountable and motivated throughout your fasting journey.

I understand that we are trapped in the same routine for years and think we cannot beat this cycle!

Do Not Worry; I Have Got Your Back!

This practical and informative book is best for women who haven't tried fasting before. It also has research-backed facts and hands-on knowledge to help you adopt a lifestyle that makes you healthy once again.

So, why wait?

I believe age is just a number; you can be fast, fit, and fabulous at any age. Are you ready to join me on this journey to healthy aging? Let's delve deep and discover the keys to becoming a better version of yourself!

Chapter 1

Aging Gracefully: Understanding Intermittent Fasting for Women Over 50 and 60

Considering fast as a treatment for aging, obesity, and type 2 disease, it mostly gets the same eye-rolling response. Starvation? What's your answer to getting fit and healthy? Are you planning to starve people? No. That's not all!

I am not asking people to starve; I am asking them to fast. It is an entirely different concept. In contrast, starvation is abstention from eating. It is neither controlled nor deliberate.

When people starve, they don't know where and when they will get their next meal. It is mainly done in times of famine or when food is scarce. Fasting is a voluntary abstention from eating for health, spiritual or other reasons. In this case, the food is available, but you do not eat it.

Fasting is not starvation. It is a spiritual discipline that has physical benefits.

-Jentezen Franklin

Fasting and starving have opposite meanings. These two should always be distinct; the terms should not be used interchangeably.

We have established the meaning of "Fasting" and how it differentiates from starvation. Let's go deep into the world of fasting, how it started, and how it has evolved in the 21st century.

Intermittent Fasting – An Ancient Idea - A Modern Concept!

Intermittent fasting has been around for thousands of years. It was practiced by many ancient civilizations, like the Greeks and Romans, as well as ancient hunter-gatherers.

It is hard to pinpoint an exact origin for intermittent fasting, but the idea that you would go through periods where you ate very little or nothing at all was in circulation for a very long time.

It wasn't until the last few decades that intermittent fasting became an increasingly popular idea, especially among those looking to lose weight and improve their overall health.

Intermittent fasting allows your body to burn off excess fat and calories naturally. With a regular diet, you will probably not be able to get snap results.

When fasting, your stomach does not have to process your food. This means that the body will work on burning off the fat stored in the body. As the body continuously burns the fat, you will lose weight quickly.

Recently, there has been a resurgence in the popularity of fasting. People are living busy lives, and with easy access to unhealthy food options, it seems challenging to maintain a healthy diet. With the help of intermittent fasting, one can take control of their health without sacrificing their lifestyle or time.

With IF, you will not have to drastically change your eating habits or keep yourself away from food all the time. You merely need to adjust when and how you eat.

I believe incorporating this regime into one's life is easier than starvation or exercise. With fasting, you can achieve your health goals easily.

Women over the age of 50 and 60 can benefit a lot from intermittent fasting. This demographic group often struggles to find a proper diet to keep their energy level full as they go through different metabolic changes.

Intermittent Fasting can help them restrict their diet and reduce cravings, so they can easily stick to a healthy diet plan and live a fabulous life.

By naturally allowing your body to burn fat stored for energy, intermittent fasting can help you lose weight quickly and safely. It is also a great way to take control of your health without making major lifestyle changes.

Is Intermittent Fasting Beneficial for Women Over 50?

Intermittent Fasting has been gaining traction worldwide due to its subtle benefits and easy approach. In this dietary approach, one has to adopt an eating pattern that involves an alternating pattern of eating and fasting. Studies show that it offers many benefits for people of all ages. But the question still remains: Does it offer the same benefits for a 50-year-old? Is it safe to practice fasting when you are in this demographic and may be battling some age-related issues?

The answer is yes. IF can be beneficial for women over 50, but it needs to be kept in mind that you need to approach this with caution and work with your healthcare professional to ensure that you are doing everything correctly.

Three main benefits that a woman over 50 can procure from fasting are:

- Weight Loss
- Improved Insulin Sensitivity
- Reduce Inflammation

Weight loss is one of the benefits that one can incur by practicing fasting. As we age, we have to deal with a slow metabolism, which makes it extremely difficult to maintain a healthy weight.

You will learn more about the diet choices and other benefits women over 50 can incur in Chapter 4. With this dietary approach, you can kickstart your weight loss by promoting fat-burning and reducing overall calorie intake.

Furthermore, women over 50 can enjoy improved insulin sensitivity with the help of IF. When we reach 50, our bodies become more prone to insulin resistance, leading to many health issues, such as type 2 diabetes. With regular fasting, you will be able to prevent or manage diabetes, and it is also known to cater to other metabolic diseases.

Inflammation reduction is also one of the benefits you get when you practice intermittent fasting. Inflammation can lead to severe health issues in older adults and can be the root cause of many chronic health conditions.

Limiting your food intake and promoting the production of anti-inflammatory compounds will allow you to see positive results in just a few days.

That being said, you need to understand that your body is going through different hormonal changes, and the intermittent fasting schedule must be adjusted accordingly.

For example, starting with 12-14 hours fast is beneficial to help your body acclimate to the new eating habits.

Myths about Intermittent Fasting

Intermittent fasting (IF) has gained popularity in recent years, and while it has been associated with various health benefits, there are also some myths and misconceptions surrounding it. It's essential to separate fact from fiction. Here are some common myths about intermittent fasting:

1) Intermittent fasting is a diet

Reality: Intermittent fasting is more of an eating pattern than a specific diet. It doesn't dictate what foods to eat but focuses on when to eat.

2) Skipping breakfast is compulsory to practice intermittent fasting

Reality: There are different methods of intermittent fasting, and not all require skipping breakfast. Some methods involve shortening the eating window or fasting for specific hours during the day.

3) Anything can be eaten during the eating window and you can still lose weight

Reality: While intermittent fasting doesn't prescribe specific foods, the quality of your diet still matters. Consuming nutrient-dense, whole foods is generally recommended for overall health and weight management.

4) Intermittent fasting slows down your metabolism

Reality: Some studies suggest that intermittent fasting may have a minor impact on metabolism, but it doesn't necessarily lead to a significant slowdown. In fact, some people may experience an increase in metabolic rate.

5) Intermittent fasting is only about weight loss

Reality: While weight loss is a common goal, intermittent fasting has been associated with other health benefits, including improved insulin sensitivity, better heart health, and potential longevity benefits.

6) It is not suitable for women

Reality: Intermittent fasting can be safe and effective for women, but individual responses may vary. It's important for women to pay attention to their bodies and adjust the fasting approach as needed.

7) Fasting for longer periods is always better

Reality: Longer fasting periods may not be suitable for everyone. The effectiveness of intermittent fasting depends on individual factors, and some people may see benefits with shorter fasting windows.

8) Intermittent fasting often leads to muscle loss

Reality: When done correctly, intermittent fasting is not likely to cause muscle loss. Adequate protein intake and resistance training can help preserve muscle mass during fasting periods.

9) It is only suitable for young and healthy individuals

Reality: While some studies have primarily focused on younger populations, there is evidence suggesting potential benefits for older adults and individuals with certain health conditions. However, consulting with a healthcare professional is advised before starting any fasting regimen.

10) Intermittent fasting works the same for everyone

Reality: Individual responses to intermittent fasting can vary. Factors such as age, sex, genetics, and overall health may influence how someone responds to this eating pattern.

It's important to approach intermittent fasting with a balanced and informed perspective, considering individual health conditions and consulting with healthcare professionals if needed.

How Intermittent Fasting Works on Body?

There is a growing body of scientific research exploring the effects of intermittent fasting on the body, and several mechanisms have been proposed to explain its impact. It's important to note that while many studies have shown promising results, research on intermittent fasting is still evolving, and individual responses can vary. Here are some key scientific aspects of how intermittent fasting may work on the body:

1) Intermittent fasting may improve **insulin sensitivity**, helping the body use insulin more effectively to regulate blood sugar levels. This can be particularly beneficial for individuals at risk of insulin resistance and type 2 diabetes.
2) Fasting periods can lead to **changes in the levels of various hormones**. For example, fasting triggers a decrease in insulin levels, allowing the body to shift from using glucose as the primary energy source to utilizing stored fat. Growth hormone levels may also increase during fasting, potentially contributing to fat breakdown and muscle preservation.
3) During fasting, the body may initiate a process called **autophagy**, which involves the removal of damaged cells and cellular components. This cellular repair mechanism is believed to have potential benefits for longevity and overall cell health.
4) Intermittent fasting may influence **gene expression and cellular adaptation**. Some studies suggest that fasting can activate genes associated with improved metabolism, stress resistance, and longevity.
5) Fasting may enhance **mitochondrial function**, the energy-producing units within cells. Improved mitochondrial function is associated with increased energy production and better cellular health.

6) Chronic inflammation is linked to various health conditions, including cardiovascular disease and metabolic disorders. Intermittent fasting has been shown to **reduce markers of inflammation**, potentially contributing to better overall health.
7) Intermittent fasting can create a **caloric deficit**, leading to weight loss. Additionally, during fasting periods, the body may increase fat oxidation as it utilizes stored fat for energy.
8) Fasting has been associated with potential cognitive benefits. It may stimulate the **production of brain-derived neurotrophic factor (BDNF),** a protein that supports brain health, learning, and memory.
9) Some studies suggest that intermittent fasting can **improve lipid profiles** by reducing levels of triglycerides and increasing levels of high-density lipoprotein (HDL) cholesterol.
10) Intermittent fasting may positively influence the **gut microbiota**, promoting a more diverse and balanced microbial community. A healthy gut microbiome is associated with various aspects of overall health.

Science Behind Intermittent Fasting for Women

Intermittent fasting is considered one of the best dietary tools for women. The main reason behind its success is its ability to regulate hormones and improve metabolism.

Millions have practiced this method, and studies show that it positively affects almost every part of the human body.

Let's look at some areas that benefit from this dieting method.

Kidneys

You can enjoy improved kidney function with the help of IF. It reduces the risk of kidney diseases and lowers blood pressure, which affects your kidneys' overall health. Intermittent fasting may have protective effects on the kidneys by reducing inflammation and oxidative stress. These benefits may contribute to a lower risk of kidney disease.

Gut

Intermittent fasting promotes healthy bacteria growth and improves overall digestion. Normalizing hormones such as leptin and ghrelin will enhance digestion, fat storage, and bowel movements.

Muscles

Intermittent fasting (IF) has been found to offer a range of benefits to women, particularly in terms of fat loss and muscle gain. It can regulate the production of IGF-1(insulin-like growth factor 1), which helps in muscle development and growth.

Brain

Intermittent fasting is linked to improved cognitive performance, potentially due to increased insulin sensitivity, less inflammation, and improved blood sugar balance. You will also see improvement in mental clarity. Women over 50 and 60 can see a reduction of stress hormones and enjoy overall brain health with IF. Intermittent fasting may promote brain health and protect against neurodegenerative diseases by supporting the production of brain-derived neurotrophic factor (BDNF), a protein associated with cognitive function and memory.

IF has been linked to reduced inflammation in the brain, which may contribute to a lower risk of neuroinflammatory conditions.

Heart

Cholesterol and insulin sensitivity are some of the primary issues older women face. Studies show that intermittent fasting is known to reduce bad cholesterol and triglycerides. It also impacts insulin production and lowers the risk of heart disease. Intermittent fasting may have positive effects on cardiovascular health by improving lipid profiles, reducing blood pressure, and enhancing insulin sensitivity, all of which contribute to a lower risk of heart disease.

Immune System

The anti-inflammatory effects and ability to control hormones improve the overall immune system function. It also reduces the risk of certain diseases and can help your body fight infections.

Hormones

Hormonal balance is very important for women over 50 and 60. A small change in the hormonal balance can lead to increased fat storage in the body, loss of appetite, and increased stress. IF can help regulate hormonal production, which ensures a better life after 50 and 60.

Pancreas

The pancreatic function is improved with the help of Intermittent fasting. With constant fasting, you will see reduced inflammation in the pancreatic area. IF can improve insulin sensitivity, potentially reducing the risk of insulin resistance and type 2 diabetes. Fasting periods help regulate blood sugar levels by enhancing the body's response to insulin.

Skin

One of the key benefits that women over 50 and 60 can get from IF is improved skin quality. The anti-inflammatory effects of fasting can positively contribute to skin issues such as acne and scars. It also promotes collagen production, thus helping keep the skin youthful and healthy.

Your organs will surely feel the effects of fasting, and it will make you feel rejuvenated and refreshed in your old age. You need to understand how IF benefits each body part, and in this way, you can use this tool to improve your overall health and well-being.

Liver

Intermittent fasting promotes the breakdown of stored fats in the liver, reducing the risk of non-alcoholic fatty liver disease (NAFLD) and improving liver function.

Fasting periods may stimulate autophagy, a process that helps remove damaged cells and cellular components, contributing to liver detoxification.

Endocrine System

IF can influence the endocrine system, leading to changes in hormone levels such as increased growth hormone release. These hormonal changes may contribute to improved metabolic health.

Adipose Tissue

Intermittent fasting creates a caloric deficit, which can contribute to weight loss. Fasting periods promote the utilization of stored fat for energy, aiding in fat loss.

Gastrointestinal System

IF may positively impact the gut microbiota, promoting a more diverse and balanced microbial community. A healthy gut microbiome is associated with various aspects of digestive health. It's important to note that while fasting has been associated with various health benefits, including those related to organ function, individual responses can vary.

Additionally, the duration and type of fasting may influence outcomes. Before starting any fasting regimen, individuals are advised to consult with healthcare professionals, especially if they have pre-existing medical conditions or concerns.

Relation between Body Metabolism and Fasting

The relationship between metabolism and fasting is complex and can vary depending on the individual, the duration of fasting, and other factors. Here are some key points to understand the connection between metabolism and fasting:

1) Effects on Hormones

Fasting can influence hormone levels, including insulin, ghrelin, and leptin. Insulin sensitivity may improve during fasting, which can have positive effects on overall metabolic health. Ghrelin and leptin, hormones related to hunger and satiety, can also be influenced by fasting.

2) Impact on Resting Metabolic Rate (RMR)

Short-term fasting may have a minimal effect on resting metabolic rate. Some studies suggest that there might be a slight decrease in RMR during fasting, but this change is generally not significant and is often compensated by other metabolic adaptations.

3) Muscle Preservation

Fasting is generally not associated with significant muscle loss, especially if the individual maintains an adequate protein intake and engages in resistance training. The body tends to prioritize fat stores over muscle tissue during short-term fasting.

4) Metabolic Flexibility

Fasting promotes metabolic flexibility, allowing the body to efficiently switch between using glucose and fatty acids for energy. This adaptability is considered a positive aspect of fasting and may contribute to improved overall metabolic health.

5) Caloric Restriction vs. Fasting

It's important to distinguish between caloric restriction and fasting. While both involve a reduction in calorie intake, fasting typically involves specific time periods without food, whereas caloric restriction usually implies a general reduction in daily calorie intake.

6) Individual Variability

Individual responses to fasting can vary based on factors such as age, sex, genetics, and overall health. What works well for one person may not be suitable for another, so it's essential to consider individual differences when exploring fasting approaches.

7) Adaptation to Fasting

The body can adapt to fasting by increasing the utilization of alternative energy sources, such as ketones derived from fat breakdown. During fasting, insulin levels decrease, prompting the body to shift from using glucose as the primary energy source to utilizing stored fats.

8) Long-term Effects

Long-term intermittent fasting has been associated with potential improvements in metabolic markers, such as insulin sensitivity and lipid profiles. However, more research is needed to understand the sustained effects and potential benefits or drawbacks of prolonged fasting.

In summary, fasting can influence various aspects of metabolism, and the effects may depend on the duration and type of fasting, as well as individual characteristics. Short-term fasting is generally well-tolerated and may have positive effects on metabolic health, but it's crucial to approach fasting with a balanced and informed perspective, considering individual needs and consulting with healthcare professionals if necessary.

I Have Crossed 60. Should I Fast?

If you are older than 60, you might be wondering if fasting is an effective way to improve your health. While fasting has many benefits for women, such as reduced inflammation, weight loss, and improved blood sugar control, it's imperative to approach this dietary regime with caution under the guidance of a healthcare professional. Intermittent fasting can have a range of benefits for women over 60, including:

Blood Sugar Control: Women over 60 are at a higher risk of type 2 diabetes. With the help of fasting, you can reduce your blood sugar level and minimize the risk of such diseases.

Fighting Heart Diseases: Fasting can help women over 60 control their weight, and subsequently, it will help to reduce the risk of chronic conditions such as arthritis and heart diseases.

Reduce Inflammation: Fasting has been shown to reduce inflammation in the body, which can help prevent chronic conditions such as heart disease, cancer, and Alzheimer's.

Risks Of Fasting for Women Over 60

While studying intermittent fasting, I mostly found the benefits associated with fasting, and no one was ready to address the potential risks related to this dietary regime. Women older than 60 are more prone to heart diseases, and when you are fasting, you should be aware of the potential risk.

Some issues that you can face when fasting are:

- Electrolyte imbalance
- Dehydration
- Low blood sugar

Electrolyte imbalance: Fasting can disrupt the balance of electrolytes in the body, leading to complications such as muscle weakness, irregular heartbeat, and fatigue. This is particularly concerning for older women, as electrolyte imbalances can exacerbate existing health conditions.

Dehydration: Older adults are already at a higher risk of dehydration due to age-related changes in thirst perception and kidney function. Fasting can further exacerbate this risk, especially if adequate fluid intake is not maintained during fasting periods.

Low blood sugar: Fasting can cause fluctuations in blood sugar levels, which may be particularly problematic for older women with diabetes or insulin resistance. Low blood sugar levels can lead to symptoms such as dizziness, weakness, confusion, and in severe cases, loss of consciousness.

The benefits and risks associated with fasting for women over 60 are described in Chapter 5.

You need to keep yourself safe while trying this health regime. You need to ensure adequate nutrition during the fasting periods. Make sure to eat a healthy diet to give the body all the nutrients it needs.

Intermittent Fasting Do's and Don'ts

IF is a widespread approach to fight obesity and other chronic issues. Like other diets and lifestyle changes, there are certain do's and don'ts that you must follow to ensure success and safety.

In this section, I will explore the key tips that will help you get the most out of your intermittent fasting.

Do's

Focus on nutrient-dense food

When you are breaking the fast, you need to focus on eating nutrient-dense foods that boost your body's energy.

Start Slowly

If you are not familiar with the concept of fasting and trying it for the first time, it is best to start slowly and gradually increase the length of your fasting periods.

Listen to your body

Not everyone has the same immunity level, and as discussed before, a fasting regime should be tailored to your body.

You need to pay attention to how your body feels during the fast, which will help you adjust the schedule.

Keep Yourself Hydrated

It is best to incorporate water and non-calorie beverages in your fasting routine. It will help you stay hydrated and improve organ function.

Consult with a healthcare professional

Before you incorporate the fasting regime into your life, you must ensure that you discuss it with your doctor. They can access your medical records and advise you on how to fast safely without compromising your health.

<u>Don'ts</u>

Overindulge when breaking the fast

It might be tempting to indulge in unhealthy food when breaking the fast. Focusing on nutrient-rich food such as minerals, lean proteins, and healthy carbs is wise.

Push yourself too hard

As we age, our bodies become less resilient. So, it would help if you avoid pushing yourself too hard during the fasting sessions.

Ignore signs of discomfort

It would be best to immediately act upon the signs of discomfort you feel during fasting. Some health concerns can be weakness, rapid heart rate, or dizziness. You need to seek medical attention and adjust your fasting approach as needed.

Neglect other aspects of a healthy lifestyle

You need to understand that fasting is just a single aspect of a healthy lifestyle. You must also prioritize adequate sleep, stress management, and exercise to maintain wellness and health.

Obsess over the clock

It would help if you did not obsess over fasting. It is good to listen to your body's cues and be flexible when you are fasting.

Don't skip meals without a plan

Intermittent fasting doesn't mean skipping meals randomly. It's essential for women over 60 to have a well-structured fasting schedule that aligns with their nutritional needs and health goals. Consult with a healthcare provider or a nutritionist to develop a fasting plan tailored to your specific needs and circumstances.

Don't neglect hydration

Older adults are more prone to dehydration, and fasting can further increase this risk. Make sure to drink plenty of water and other hydrating fluids during non-fasting periods to maintain optimal hydration levels.

Should I seek Medical Attention Before Fasting at This Age?

Yes, seeking medical attention before you delve into the world of intermittent fasting is a wise idea. As we get older, our bodies react differently to different types of diets and fasting schedules. A medical practitioner will help you understand how fasting can affect your body.

It would be best to discuss any underlying health conditions you have with your healthcare professional. In this way, your doctor can provide an appropriate fasting plan tailored to your health needs.

Hershel can also recommend the modifications you can make in your fasting approach based on age and health status. They can tell you about the nutrient-rich food to incorporate into your diet to support your overall health.

I recommend seeking medical attention before you plan to start the fasting routine. You must ensure you take all the necessary precautions to practice IF safely.

Take a look at the table given below and discuss all these topics when seeking medical attention:

Headings	Information to include
Medical History	Any pre-existing medical conditions or chronic illnesses.
Medications	List of medications you are currently taking.
Allergies	Any known allergies to medications, foods, or other substances.
Previous Fasting Experience	Details of any previous fasting attempts or experiences.
Fasting Plan	The type of fasting you intend to follow (e.g., intermittent fasting, extended fasting) and its duration.
Exercise Routine	Description of your current exercise routine, including any high-intensity or strenuous activities.
Dietary Considerations	Any dietary restrictions, intolerances, or specific food preferences.
Concerns or Questions	Do you have any specific concerns or questions regarding fasting, exercise, or yoga at your age?
Desired Outcome	Explain your goals or desired outcome from incorporating fasting, exercise, and yoga into your routine.

Preferred Contact Method	How do you prefer to receive feedback or recommendations from the healthcare professional (e.g., in-person appointment, phone call, email)?

Chapter 2

The 6 Intermittent Fasting Methods You Need to Try Now!

What do you mean by different fasting regimes? Isn't fasting a singular concept? Do I need to learn about different fasting methods to get positive results? I was bombarded with such questions when I tried explaining fasting to my mom.

Do not worry, I will explain all while keeping things light and fun.

In the first chapter, we have covered the introduction and importance of intermittent fasting. From improving brain function to reducing inflammation, IF has been linked to many positive outcomes. But with so many different approaches to intermittent fasting, it is difficult to decide which regime to follow.

Certainly! Exploring the variety of fasting regimes can offer insights into which approach aligns best with individual preferences, lifestyles, and health goals.

"Fasting cleanses the soul, raises the mind, subjects one's flesh to the spirit, renders the heart contrite and humble, scatters the clouds of concupiscence, and quenches the fire of lust, and kindles the true light of chastity." - St. Augustine.

In this chapter, we will explore six famous IF strategies. By understanding benefits and drawbacks of each of these benefits, you can choose the one that works best for you.

The most prominent types of intermittent fasting are:

- The 16:8 Method
- The warrior diets
- Time-restricted fasting
- The 5:2 Diet
- Alternate-day fasting
- Eat stop eat

Each fasting regime offers unique benefits and challenges, and there is no one-size-fits-all approach. It's essential to experiment with different methods and find what works best for individual preferences, health goals, and lifestyles.

16/8 Intermittent Fasting Method

The 16:8 fasting is one of the most favored methods for losing weight. Women over 50 can practice this method and see results in a few weeks. It is also known as time-restricted fasting.

In this method, a person fasts for 16 straight hours and restricts eating for 8 hours.

There are different strategies by which you can approach this. Some people miss breakfast and restrict eating from 12 pm to 8 pm. Other people choose to miss supper. In this way, they could eat from 9 am to 5 pm every day.

In this technique, you will have the option to eat the main meal of the day. You can adjust your eating time if you do not want to disrupt your calorie intake or skip a meal. For example, you can eat breakfast at 10 am, lunch at 1.30 pm, and dinner at 5:30 pm.

So, in this manner, you will be able to finish all your meals in the 8-hour eating window.

Fasting limits the person from eating for the remaining 16 hours of thc day. Other diet plans have a rigid set of rules and regulations, while the 16/8 process is more flexible and is based on the time-restricted feeding method.

Pros

This method is easy to execute and can help people facing issues with blood pressure. Limiting the food intake will help women over 50 and 60 lose weight and lower their blood pressure.

A review study showcased that those who did little aerobic exercise while practicing the 16/8 method maintained their muscle mass while reducing body fat. Apart from this, another study shows improved cholesterol levels and reduced risk of heart disease in those who practiced this method for more than two months.

Cons

While this is one of the safest ways to practice intermittent fasting, if you approach this without consultation with your doctor, it may lead to weakness and fatigue. It is wise to listen to the body's signals when practicing this regime. If you are facing severe headaches or sleep issues, it is best to consult with your doctor.

The Warrior Diets

This fasting regime is termed the warrior diet because it follows the ancient warriors' eating patterns. This diet was created in 2001 and is more intense than the 16:8 method. It is also termed as the 20:4 method.

Women over 50 should not immediately jump into this regime. In this diet, you will just have a 4-hour eating window and eat small quantities of food for the next 20 hours. The fasting experts recommend eating hard-boiled eggs during the fasting period.

Apart from this, you can also eat raw fruits and drink fluids that have no calories. Studies reveal that a time-restricted diet can inhibit diabetes and other chronic diseases.

As discussed earlier, adopting a warrior diet can be fairly difficult, as the time for significant calorie intake is just 4 hours. On the other hand, choosing a 4-hour eating window is also a considerable problem. Excessive eating during the eating window can also lead to many health problems, such as bloating and heart burn.

Pros

This intermittent fasting regime is strict and helps to reduce body fat. This will ultimately help women over 50 reduce their weight.

On the plus side, a study revealed that the 20:4 diet is linked with improved brain health and cognitive function. It helps shield the body against Alzheimer's and other brain issues. Like other intermittent fasting techniques, this method reduces the risk of type 2 diabetes.

Cons

The longer fasting period in the 20:4 diet can lead to sustainability issues. Women over 50 may start this diet and continue it for a couple of days, but you need to understand that without consistency, you will not be able to see the desired results.

Another problem with this fasting regime is the issue of binge eating. With a few hours to complete your daily calorie intake, you must eat more than 90% of your daily food during this time. Apart from this, fatigue, dizziness, and low blood sugar are common problems encountered during the first days of this regime.

Time-restricted fasting

In time-restricted fasting, you get to choose the feeding window every day. You must select a 14 or 16-hour fasting window and leave 8 hours for eating. It is recommended for women over 50 to not exceed the 14-hour fasting window in the first month due to hormonal issues.

During fasting, women over 50 can only drink water to stay hydrated. TRE (time-restricted eating) might not work for everybody, and a person needs to follow this diet longer to see results. This fasting regime can also help build muscle mass and reduce inflammation. TRE is best for women looking to control their calorie intake.

Pros

The time-restricted diet reduces weight, improves heart health, and lowers blood sugar levels. Bad cholesterol increases the risk of heart disease. When you practice TRE, you will see an increase in good cholesterol, impacting your heart health. Adding exercise to this diet can help you build endurance.

Cons

As this method is flexible, women tend to miss days when they have to fast. This can lead to breaking the entire cycle and getting no results.

The 5:2 Diet

The 5:2 method entails consuming a normal number of calories for five days a week and then reducing the calorie consumption to 500-600 calories for the remaining two days. This is also known as the fast diet. It is one of the simple and direct intermittent fasting plans. You normally eat for five days but do not eat unhealthy or fried items. Then, you drop the calorie consumption to one-quarter of what you ate the entire week. So, for instance, if you eat 2000 calories on the normal days, you will eat just 500 calories in the remaining 2 days.

This fasting regime is especially helpful for people who have type 2 diabetes. They can easily work on their weight loss without having an issue. There is no limitation on the days you select for eating normally. You get a free pass to eat whatever you want. The 5:2 diet can be efficient, but it is not meant for everybody.

Pros

One of the best things about this diet plan is that no food item is off limit and you can eat whatever you want. Additionally, you get to choose the fasting days.

Cons

During the two days, if you limit your food intake, you might have trouble sleeping and experience irritable behavior. Apart from this, reducing the calorie intake to one-quarter of your normal routine can cause constipation.

Eat - Stop - Eat

Eat, stop, eat is an effective intermittent fasting technique for women over 50. It is a method of intermittent fasting that involves two fasts per week. The time span of the fast is 24 hours, and they are non-consecutive. It means that you will intake just one meal two days a week. This meal could be breakfast, lunch or dinner according to your wish.

The eat-stop-eat method reduces your caloric intake. When you intake no food for 24 hours, your calorie intake decreases. According to research, just one 24-hour fast lowers 10% of calories in a person.

This technique helps to shift your metabolism into fat-burning mode. When you eat throughout the day, the body obtains the energy it requires from the food you eat. You usually eat breakfast, lunch, and dinner, but when you fast, the body gets energy from the stored glucose of the muscles.

Once all the glucose is used up, the body shifts to burning fat for energy. Ketosis is a term used for this metabolic shift. It specifically targets fat cells.

Pros

There are various benefits of the stop-eat IF method, such as it helps to reduce inflammation. Chronic inflammation puts women over 50 at greater risk for serious health problems. This method improves inflammatory markers and reduces the risk of severe health issues.

Cardiovascular health is greatly enhanced by this method. It helps control cholesterol levels and lowers blood pressure, improving heart health. Research shows that fasting is ideal for improving glycemic control and lowering insulin resistance.

It ultimately reduces the risk of type 2 diabetes. Intermittent fasting creates hormonal shifts that will enhance our health. It helps to produce a high level of norepinephrine.

Cons

Fruits and vegetables consist of a significant amount of water. Fasting for 24 hours increases the risk of dehydration. Dehydration is observed in active people.

Constipation is another problem that you can face while intermittent fasting. Ideally, you need 25-35 g of fiber a day. Achieving your fiber goal can be difficult during fasting. The low fiber in the body increases the risk of constipation.

Some people develop eating disorders from long-term fasting. Long fasting hours can make you nutrient-deficient.

Alternate-Day Fasting

The alternate-day fasting method is the same as the name; you fast on alternate days. One day, you restrict your calorie intake, and the other day, you feast as much as you like, in any amount.

Fasting days can be a strict version when you don't intake any calories at all. On the contrary, the modified version allows you to eat up 25% of your energy needs, which is around 500 calories.

During the modified version of alternate-day fasting, you can eat meals that are either home-cooked or packaged. Water, unsweetened tea, and black coffee are also allowed at any time of day. Foods high in fiber and proteins will help you cope with hunger. Soups help to fill up the stomach without adding many calories.

Pros

Alternate-day fasting dramatically helps in losing weight. People cut back on their meals to lose weight. This is known as caloric restriction. There is a problem with the caloric restriction that requires reducing energy intake every day.

This can stimulate cravings and hunger. The alternate-day fasting creates a calorie deficit in a sustainable and easy way. Eating less every other day creates enough calorie deficit over time that causes weight loss.

Alternate-day fasting helps to reduce cholesterol, improves heart health, and reduces the risk of diabetes.

Cons

The common problems arising from alternate-day fasting are irritability, hunger, constipation, dizziness, bad breath, and weakness. In rare cases, the bone mineral density is also decreased.

Religious Fasting

Religious fasting is a practice observed by many individuals around the world as part of their faith traditions. Fasting in a religious context often involves abstaining from certain foods, drinks, or activities for a specific period. Different religions have distinct fasting practices, each serving unique spiritual, cultural, or historical purposes.

Muslims observe fasting during the month of Ramadan, the ninth month of the Islamic lunar calendar. From dawn to sunset, practitioners abstain from food, drink, smoking, and sinful behavior. The fast is broken with a meal called iftar at sunset. Fasting during Ramadan is one of the Five Pillars of Islam.

Yom Kippur, the Day of Atonement, is observed with a 25-hour fast by Jewish individuals. Tisha B'Av is another day of mourning that involves fasting. During these fasts, participants abstain from food, drink, and other physical needs.

In Christianity, Lent is a period of 40 days leading up to Easter, commemorating the 40 days Jesus spent fasting in the desert. Many Christians choose to fast or give up certain luxuries during this time, with fasting often involving abstaining from meat on Fridays.

In Hinduism, fasting is often observed on specific days, such as Ekadashi, which occurs twice a month. Navaratri, a festival lasting nine nights, involves fasting, prayer, and celebration. Fasting practices can vary among different sects and regions.

Buddhism includes various forms of fasting, especially during special observances and retreats. Monks often follow specific rules regarding when and what they can eat. Lay Buddhists may also practice intermittent fasting or abstain from certain foods during religious events.

Sikhs celebrate Gurpurab, the birth anniversary of Sikh Gurus, with special prayers, community service, and sometimes fasting. The practice of fasting can vary among Sikh individuals and communities.

Bahá'í adherents fast from sunrise to sunset during the Bahá'í month of Ala, which precedes the Bahá'í New Year (Naw-Rúz). Fasting during this period is considered a time of spiritual reflection and renewal.

Religious fasting goes beyond the physical act of abstaining; it is a multifaceted practice that encompasses spiritual reflection, self-control, cmpathy, and communal solidarity. The specific rules, duration, and significance of fasting vary widely among different religious traditions, reflecting the diversity of beliefs and practices worldwide.

Now that you have learned about different fasting regimes, you can easily choose which diet to follow. Remember that consultation with the doctor is extremely important before jumping into any regime.

The main aim of fasting is to be youthful and active as we age, and there are many secret benefits of fasting that you will explore as you dig deep into this book.

No matter the fasting schedule you opt for, here are some nutritional guidelines that you should take into consideration:

Nutritional Guidelines During Fasting	**Recommendations**
Caloric Intake	None Or Very Minimal Caloric Intake During Fasting Period.
Hydration	Drink Plenty of Water Throughout the Fasting Period.
Macronutrients	Prioritize Consuming Nutrient-Dense Foods During the Eating Window.
Protein	Include Adequate Protein to Support Muscle Health and Maintenance.

Carbohydrates	Focus On Complex Carbohydrates Like Whole Grains, Legumes, And Vegetables.
Fats	Incorporate Healthy Fats Like Avocados, Nuts, Seeds, And Olive Oil.
Fiber	Consume Fiber-Rich Foods to Support Digestion and Satiety.
Micronutrients	Ensure Sufficient Intake of Vitamins and Minerals Through Diverse Food Choices.
Supplements	Consider Consulting a Healthcare Professional for Guidance on Supplement Needs.

Chapter 3

13 Secrets to Stay Fast, Fit, And Fabulous At 50+

Are you facing issues with your health and looking for ways to stay fast, fit, and fabulous at 50+? After 50, It is common to see changes in the body, but one should not slow down or give up on the wellness goals.

> *"Fasting is the practice of sacrifice in the most noble sense of the word. It's a sacrifice that is made for a higher purpose." - Jason Fung.*

In this chapter, I will tell you 13 proven and practical strategies to help your physical and mental well-being as you age.

From nutrition to stress management and self-care, you will learn to stay on track with your happiness and health goals. Intermittent Fasting can help in all ages, but if you want to get the best out of your golden years. Explore and implement these strategies and see the result for yourself!

With the right fasting routine, mindset, and habits, you can feel energized and confident in your 50s, 60s, and beyond.

- Secret 1: Make Intermittent Fasting a Lifestyle
- Secret 2: Start Slow and Work Your Way Up
- Secret 3: Prioritize Protein
- Secret 4: Stay Hydrated
- Secret 5: Practice Mindful Eating
- Secret 6: Experiment with Different Fasting Protocols
- Secret 7: Get Enough Sleep
- Secret 8: Manage Stress
- Secret 9: Mind Your Eating Windows
- Secret 10: Be Patient and Persistent
- Secret 11: Practice Self-Care
- Secret 12: Seek Support from Others
- Secret 13: Stay Educated and Curious about the Latest Research

Secret 1: Make Intermittent Fasting a Lifestyle

It would help if you did not take intermittent fasting as a diet but consider it a lifestyle. If you plan to reap the benefits of IF, you must commit to it as a long-term lifestyle change. Embracing the idea of fasting regularly and making it a part of your daily routine can help you quickly envision your health goals.

Numerous research studies highlight the importance of intermittent fasting. You will get many health benefits, such as improved blood sugar levels, decreased inflammation, and reduced risk of chronic diseases like cancer and arthritis. You must understand that you can only benefit from intermittent fasting if you consistently stick to it.

Let's say you have been fasting for a few weeks, and then there is a need to travel, and you decide to break the fast earlier than usual. This is fine as a one-time occurrence, but if you start finding excuses to break the fast earlier every time, you will not be able to see the benefits of fasting. You need to plan ahead and stick to your fasting habits even when you need to travel or go to any social event.

Making intermittent fasting a lifestyle change can take time and effort, but the rewards are well worth it. By committing to a regular fasting routine, you can achieve better health and wellness as you age and feel more in control of your eating habits. So, make it a priority to embrace intermittent fasting as a long-term lifestyle change, and watch as the benefits start to pile up over time.

Secret 2: Start Slow and Work Your Way Up

If you are not used to going without food for a longer time, then intermittent fasting can be challenging. You need to make sure that you start slow and gradually work your way up to longer fasts. Gradual adjustments to intermittent fasting are seen as more sustainable and effective in the long run.

According to the Journal of the Academy of Nutrition and Dietetics, the participants who gradually increased their fast time achieved better weight loss and improved metabolism results than those who started with longer fasting right away.

If you are new to intermittent fasting, you should aim for a 16:8 fasting protocol. I understand fasting for 16 hours and only having an 8-hour eating window seems difficult. A simple approach to tackle this is starting with a 12-hour fast and gradually adding an hour to your fasting regime.

In this way, your body will get used to fasting, and you will not always feel tired or hungry. Gradually adding hours to the fasting routine will open ways for new good habits in your life. As your body feels rejuvenated, you will feel motivated to take up good things for your soul and body. So, do not just go straight into a brutal fasting regime; start slow and watch your body adapt to your routine.

Secret 3: Prioritize Protein

A balanced diet is what keeps us healthy. If you are more than 50 and start practicing intermittent fasting, you need to make sure that you have a protein-rich diet. Protein helps in supporting muscle repair and growth. Different studies also showcase that eating a high-protein diet is beneficial for weight maintenance and helps reduce the risk of chronic diseases such as type 2 diabetes.

Suppose you are practicing intermittent fasting and only have a meal window of 8 hours. It is best to prioritize protein-rich foods during this time.

Some food items that you should prioritize are lean meat, nuts, eggs, and legumes. They will help you feel fuller and more satisfied.

Secret 4: Stay Hydrated

Regardless of your age group, keeping track of your water intake is best. Dehydration can cause different issues in the human body. Staying hydrated is especially imperative when you are practicing intermittent fasting. Drinking abundant water supports healthy digestion and helps fight obesity while reducing hunger.

Different research depicts the importance of drinking water before a meal. For instance, it is reported that drinking water before a meal can increase the feeling of fullness and reduce hunger. A low-calorie diet with increased water intake is a successful strategy for women over 50 who are looking to shed weight.

When you are fasting, it is vital to stay hydrated. You should aim for at least 8-10 glasses of water daily. Remember that other beverages like coffee and herbal tea can also contribute to your daily fluid intake. Be careful about extra sugar and calories in certain drinks, as these can disrupt your fasting periods and potentially lead to weight gain.

Secret 5: Practice Mindful Eating

Mindful eating is the phenomenon of being fully engaged and mentally present during meals. You need to focus on the textures and flavors of the food and listen to the body's signals. Practicing mindful eating is helpful during fasting because it can help avoid overeating during the eating windows.

A study in the **IJBNPA** - International Journal of Behavioral Nutrition and Physical Activity) showcases that mindfulness-based eating helps promote healthy eating habits while reducing binge eating.

The eating windows are limited when you are practicing intermittent fasting. So, it is best to be mindful of what and how much you eat. I have found a small hack that will surely help you with this. Unwind and focus on what your goals are before you start eating. You should chew slowly, pay attention to the food, and savor each bite.

Listening to your body's fullness and hunger signals would be best. Eating faster or overeating can lead to discomfort and weight gain.

Secret 6: Experiment with Different Fasting Protocols

Many intermittent fasting protocols exist, and what works best for one person may not work for another. Experimenting with different fasting protocols is essential to find what works best for your body and lifestyle.

A study published in the International Journal of Obesity found that alternate-day fasting was an effective weight loss strategy for some individuals. In contrast, others may benefit more from time-restricted feeding.

Another study published in the Journal of Translational Medicine found that individuals following an intermittent fasting protocol that included calorie restriction and time-restricted feeding experienced greater improvements in metabolic health markers than those following either protocol alone.

Some popular protocols include time-restricted feeding, alternate-day fasting, and the 5:2 diet.

Pay attention to how your body responds to each protocol and adjust as necessary. By experimenting with different fasting protocols, you can find a sustainable approach that works best for your body and lifestyle.

Secret 7: Get Enough Sleep

We have heard this tip thousands of times, which is equally essential when practicing intermittent fasting over 50. Sleep-regulated hormones control hunger and metabolism, and proper sleep can help regulate them. A study from the Journal of Obesity found that sleep deprivation can lead to increased appetite and hunger.

You should aim for at least 7-8 hours of sleep every night and maintain this schedule. I recommend going to bed and waking up at the same time each day. This will help adjust the sleep cycle; consequently, your stomach will get signals about when to work and go into hibernation. Some tips that can help you adjust the sleep cycle are:

- Stay Away from Distractions When You Go to Bed, i.e., Cell Phone and Laptop
- Be Mindful of Your Sleep Environment
- Try Taking a Warm Bath Before Sleep
- Exercising Before Sleep Can Relax the Muscles
- Choose A Dark and Quiet Space for Sleeping

You can support healthy hormone regulation and minimize cravings and hunger by indulging in proper sleep. So, ensure that you sleep properly during the intermittent fasting routine.

Secret 8: Manage Stress

Stress is the leading cause of many mental and physical issues. It also affects our metabolism and weight. When practicing intermittent fasting, you must prioritize stress management to meet your health goals.

A study published in the journal Obesity Reviews found that chronic stress was associated with an increased risk of obesity and metabolic disorders. Another study published in the journal "Psych neuroendocrinology" found that acute stress was associated with increased levels of the hunger hormone ghrelin, which can lead to overeating.

Breathing exercises, journaling, and yoga can help minimize stress. It would help if you also made a checklist of things that affect your mood and ultimately give you anxiety. Remembering the stress triggers and fighting them can help you improve your overall mental health.

It's important to find stress management techniques that work for you and that you enjoy, so don't be afraid to try different strategies until you find what feels best.

Secret 9: Mind Your Eating Windows

When practicing intermittent fasting, you must be mindful of your eating windows to ensure you give your body the nutrients it needs to thrive.

A study published in the Journal of Nutrition found that eating a larger proportion of calories earlier in the day was associated with more significant weight loss in individuals following a weight loss program. Another study published in the Journal of Obesity found that time-restricted feeding, a type of intermittent fasting, was associated with improved metabolic health markers in individuals with prediabetes.

When practicing intermittent fasting, you must be mindful of your eating windows to ensure you get the nutrients you need to support your body.

By being mindful of your eating windows and prioritizing nutrient-dense, whole foods during these times, you can support your overall health and well-being while practicing intermittent fasting.

Secret 10: Be Patient and Persistent

As discussed in the first chapter, intermittent fasting is not a quick-fix solution. You need to understand that you might see results after a few weeks. Whether starting intermittent fasting for weight loss or improving cognitive function, you must stay focused and patient during the journey.

It would be best to remember that you have been eating carelessly for many years, and it might take some time for your stomach to adjust to this new reality and show results. A study from Obesity Science and Practice showcased that people who have been practicing intermittent fasting for more than 2-year have shown more remarkable persistence in their weight loss journey than those who are eating normally.

Do not expect immediate results; be prepared to face setbacks and challenges. You need to set realistic goals and focus on the long-term benefits of this dietary method. Track your progress along the way and celebrate after small accomplishments.

I have already emphasized that intermittent fasting is not a one-size-fits-all strategy. So, what might work for someone else might not have the same effect on you. It is best to experiment with different regimes to find the perfect fit for your body.

Secret 11: Practice Self-Care

Believe me when I say that self-care is one of the best things to make you feel fit and fabulous, regardless of age.

With intermittent fasting, you can improve your overall health and longevity. Exercising regularly, effective stress management, and choosing a healthy diet can help overcome many physical and mental issues.

You should choose nutrient-dense food and have a good sleeping routine to ensure you are on track to meet your overall health goals. When you face issues or setbacks practicing self-care, I advise sharing your feelings with your loved ones. They can support you and help you get back on track.

Secret 12: Seek Support from Others

When you are older than 50, your life takes different turns. You are entering the menopause stage, and most women are free from obligations such as children and work. This is when a support system can help you get your physical health on track.

Seeking support from family, friends, and an online community of like-minded people can help you excel in your intermittent fasting journey. It is best to share your goals and progress when needed. Talking about your journey can also help you get the encouragement you need to prosper.

Many people have different mindsets, and some of us thrive when cornered or judged. I am one of these people, and what I found helpful is having an accountability partner who is also practicing intermittent fasting. My accountability partner was my grandmother, who is 56 years old. She used to check on me daily and ask about my progress. This helped me stay on track and helped me forge a strong bond with her.

So, by seeking support from others, your chances of success increase tenfold, making your intermittent fasting journey fulfilling and enjoyable.

Secret 13: Stay Educated and Curious About the Latest Research

To successfully practice intermittent fasting over 50, it's important to stay informed and curious about the latest research on fasting and its potential benefits. By staying educated, you can make informed decisions about your fasting approach and ensure that you're following the most up-to-date guidelines.

Research in the field of intermittent fasting is continually evolving, and new studies are published regularly. By staying curious, you can seek out and explore the latest findings, advancements, and insights related to fasting. This can include reading scientific studies, following reputable health and nutrition sources, and staying connected with experts in the field.

By staying educated, you can better understand the potential health benefits of intermittent fasting, such as improved metabolic health, weight management, cognitive function, and longevity. You can also gain knowledge about different fasting protocols and strategies that may be specifically beneficial for individuals over 50.

Furthermore, staying educated and curious allows you to critically evaluate information and differentiate between evidence-based findings and unsubstantiated claims or trends. It empowers you to make informed choices that align with your individual health goals, preferences, and any specific considerations related to your age or health condition.

Remember, the field of nutrition and fasting research is dynamic, and there is still much to learn. By staying educated and staying curious, you can stay at the forefront of knowledge and maximize the potential benefits of intermittent fasting for your overall well-being.

Intermittent fasting is not just a diet; it is a lifestyle that you can adopt to make permanent changes in your life. You will feel younger and more energetic and will feel mental and physical changes like never before.

Keep in mind that every person has a different metabolism, and it might take some time for you to adjust to the new lifestyle. Consistency is the key to success when it comes to intermittent fasting. In the next chapter, I will help you understand how you can achieve your health goals by fasting.

Chapter 4

Shaping Women's Health: Achieve Your Health Goals by Fasting At 50

To understand the effects of fasting on women over 50, I will discuss the functionality of the reproductive system, the hormones responsible for conceiving a baby, and how fasting affects women at different ages.

"Fasting is the greatest remedy--the physician within." - Philipps Paracelsus.

Fasting affects the women's bodies in many ways. When you are fasting, it regulates the reproductive hormone called hypothalamic-pituitary-gonadal. This reproductive hormone is found in both men and women. The hypothalamus is responsible for releasing a gonadotropin-releasing hormone called "pulses." Gonadotropin-releasing hormones (GnRH) are responsible for releasing the stimulation hormone (LH) and luteinizing hormone (LH) (FSH). These two hormones in women are needed for a mature woman to conceive.

In some women, short-term fasting may change the hormonal pulses. In some cases, it is reported that skipping a single meal can put the reproductive system on alert, which is not in a state of emergency by itself. This is why, without proper consultation, intermittent fasting can cause issues for some women.

But here arises a question. Why does skipping a meal put our body in an alert form? Scientists have believed that women's body fat percentage regulated their reproductive system for many years. If the body fat percentage falls below a certain level, the hormones will get confused, and the cycle stops.

This made a lot of sense from an evolutionary perspective, but studies have shown that even if the body fat percentage falls below a certain amount, let's say 11 percent, a woman's body can still go on alert, and reproduction is possible.

How An Irregular Diet Can Work Against You

You are in a negative energy balance when you consistently consume less food than the energy you spend. You are in a state of dieting when you get into a negative energy balance. This is what many women are trying to achieve by dieting. But dieting alone cannot help with weight loss. Many factors affect a woman's hormonal balance, leading to bad eating habits and weight gain.

Negative hormonal changes can result from:

- Infection, chronic inflammation
- An excessive amount of exercise
- Poor nutrition
- Too much stress
- Not giving your body time for recovery

Intermittent Fasting and Lifetime of Females

A woman's body goes through different stages of existence that are marked by major hormonal alterations.

These changes have a major impact on psychological and physical health. They can affect digestion, reactivity to stress, metabolism, and even sleep. I have highlighted some stages of a woman's life and discussed how intermittent fasting affects her body.

Girls And Teens

Intermittent fasting is not recommended during times of intense development. Many teenagers may put themselves under many scrutinizes and social comparisons and limit their diet. This change in eating habits can affect their growth. It is advised to focus on nutritious food items. Promoting enjoyable and stress-free relationships with food is essential for teenagers.

Ovulating Women and Fasting

If you are trying to conceive, intermittent fasting may complicate things. Ovulation is affected by fasting. This means that no egg is released if you are not ovulating. Doctors and other health practitioners may recommend women lose weight before getting pregnant.

The first thing that comes to a woman's mind is dieting. But a strict dieting regime is not what you want if you plan to conceive. Most women can easily shed some pounds with good eating behaviors.

Intermittent Fasting During Pregnancy

Like adolescence and childhood, pregnancy is also an intense development period. Weight gain is natural in this stage and is seen as a symbol of stable infant growth. Women can get extremely conscious during this time. Some women are prescribed to control their weight during this period. Even if the doctor is asking to lose weight, it is not recommended for women to fast during pregnancy. A healthy diet can help women lose weight.

It would be best to focus on the nutrients rather than starving yourself. You can also boost your health and control weight with the help of yoga and minimalistic exercises.

Intermittent Fasting in Aging Females

I understand you may have been waiting for this section. But giving context to how fasting affects women of different ages will help you develop a benchmark in your mind and understand menopause in a better fashion.

Puberty, menstruation, pregnancy: A woman's body goes through many changes and feels like a rollercoaster.

Then comes the stage called menopause. This hormonal transition point changes the women's lives both physically and mentally.

After giving decades to their career, children, and other aspects of life, this is the time women can focus on themselves. You might still be busy with young adult children or looking after your parents, but this stage will give you ample time to focus on your overall health.

It is considered one of the most complicated phases in a woman's life. It is time to learn about these natural transitions and how to fast safely and live happily.

Many women are not ready for these changes and take this as a sign of defeat. It is important to remain calm and minimize the negative effects of suffering. As discussed in the last chapter, you need to seek support from your loved ones and ensure that you embrace targeted nutrition to stay active beyond 50.

Learn What Happens to The Body of a Menopausal Woman

The pre-menopausal stage, lasting from 45 to 50 years, is when women see a reduction in the production of the hormone estrogen. This is why women at this age see changes in their menstrual cycle.

During this time, women also experience subjective endocrine changes that can lead to headaches, depression, and sleep disorders. When a woman enters the actual menopause stage, the production of estrogen drastically decreases, and the range of symptoms widens.

There is also a change in the bone balance; women with increased mobilization and nutrient-deficit diets may face skeletal issues.

Although women face different changes during menopause, metabolism is affected the most. The absorption and accumulation of sugars change, and some studies also showcase the changes in the clinical values of triglycerides that can lead to high blood pressure.

The Ideal Diet for Menopause

Some studies suggest that the arrival of menopause may also come with some disorders. Doctors prescribe natural therapy or drugs with a specific diet to fight these.

Different variables come into play, and it is necessary to modify our food routine to help our bodies adapt to these changes naturally. The main problem many women face is fat accumulation in the belly region due to the drop in estrogen. Digestion is also affected by the slower intestinal function of the women.

Therefore, you need to be ready because the beginning period of menopause will be more problematic to manage. Effective distribution of nutrients can help cope with this.

How To Approach a Fasting Regime with Menopause

Women who are concerned about menopause can see positive results with intermittent fasting. A lower estrogen level in women can lead to a reduced ability to cope with stress. Add sleep disturbances, and your stress bucket fills pretty soon.

You should try intermittent fasting only if:

- Your stress level is relatively low
- Mood swings do not torment you
- You do not have any nutrient deficiency
- Your sleep quality is good

Fasting isn't for everyone, but there are different fasting regimes that you can try, and with experimentation, you can find a perfect fit for you.

Finding The Right Intermittent Fasting Routine for Women Over 50

There are different ways to get the best out of your fasting regime. It would be best to have a perfect sense of your body's needs before diving into the world of fasting. Start by keeping a food journal. Understand what you are eating and how often you eat it.

Some questions that you might need answers to are

- Do you eat late at night or like having snacks during the day?
- Do you eat lighter meals or prefer large ones that fill you up?
- Do you like protein in every meal or prefer veggies?
- Practicing light fasting to get some baseline is recommended by many dietitians. Here are a few ways to do it:
- Start by stretching the intervals between eating.
- Check what your body signals when you stop eating or increase the intervals.
- Do you feel totally fine after skipping dinner?
- Although these may initially feel uncomfortable, is the overall hunger manageable? Track yourself with curiosity and integrity. You can proceed with a gentle IF method if you feel mentally sharp and energetic.

Chapter 5

Golden Rules: Navigating Fasting for Women Over 60

Who would have thought that the "whisper" of hunger could hold the key to unlocking a golden chapter of vitality and well-being for women over 60?

"The best of all medicines is resting and fasting." - Benjamin Franklin

---

We have seen a constant rise in the popularity of Intermittent fasting among people of all ages, and many studies showcase that this dieting regime is especially beneficial for women over the age of 60.

Aging comes with many key health issues, and Intermittent fasting is one of the best ways to prevent and even prevent the effects of these issues. It will help you lead a more fulfilling and healthier life.

Women over 60 see several changes in their bodies. From a decline in metabolism, bone density, and muscle mass to being at a higher risk of health conditions such as cancer and diabetes, older women are prone to many health issues. Intermittent fasting is a widespread technique to tackle these health issues and improve overall health outcomes for women over 60.

Unlocking Health Benefits: Fasting for Women Over 60

The decline in metabolism coupled with stomach issues make it quite difficult for women over 60 to maintain a healthy weight. While some women see a reduction in muscle mass, others fight obesity. With the help of Intermittent fasting, women can see increased weight loss and improved metabolism. When IF is combined with regular exercise, positive results can be seen in less than a month.

Additionally, this dietary regime is also known to prevent diabetes and have anti-inflammatory effects on the body. Women over 60 who are at risk of heart disease, cancer, and arthritis can see positive results by practicing intermittent fasting. Apart from this, reduction in bone density is one of the main issues older women face. This can lead to osteoporosis, and intermittent fasting can help reduce the risk of such disease.

Controlling the diet also has a positive impact on insulin sensitivity. Women over 60 are at a higher risk of developing diabetes, and to fight it, you need to exercise regularly and incorporate IF in your lifestyle.

You can expect many benefits when you start practicing intermittent fasting. This dietary regime can help you maintain overall health while preventing chronic diseases. Like other dietary changes, you need to consult with your doctor about your health conditions and should take advice on how to proceed with intermittent fasting.

Considerations To Safely Navigate Fasting Over 60

Fasting offers numerous health benefits, but knowing its potential pitfalls is equally important. Taking necessary precautions to minimize the adverse effects of fasting can help you a lot in the long run.

First and foremost, I would emphasize safeguarding health through medical consultation. Your metabolism and nutritional needs change as you age, and the healthcare provider will help you understand these changes and navigate fasting easily. With access to your medical records, doctors can easily identify any potential issue that may arise when you practice intermittent fasting.

Nutrient deficiencies are one significant concern for women over 60. With slow metabolism and less nutrient absorption, prolonged fasts can exacerbate this issue. To tackle such problems, it is imperative to have a well-balanced diet of nutrient-rich food such as whole grains, lean protein, and vegetables. If you feel tired and unable to continue fasting after 60, you can also consider using supplements under a healthcare professional's guidance.

It is essential to maintain hydration during fasting periods. Dehydration can have severe effects on older women, and women over 60 should aim to drink an adequate amount of water during fasting periods. It will help support overall health and prevent complications.

Women who suffer from diabetes and hypoglycemia should take extra care when fasting. Fasting is known to lower sugar levels, and monitoring blood sugar levels regularly during fasting is advised. You must also adjust your fasting regime based on your blood sugar level. To ensure a stable blood sugar level, alternative fasting methods such as time-restricted eating are best.

The most important consideration is that women over 60 must be mindful of their medication. You can get help from your doctor to determine the best approach for using medication during fasting. You may need to adjust the fasting protocol accordingly because some medications require food intake for proper functioning.

Lastly, women over 60 must listen to their body cues and be mindful of any adverse effects of fasting. Issues such as confusion, dizziness, and weakness shall be immediately addressed. If you feel any concerning symptoms, it is imperative to break the fast and seek medical attention.

Decoding the Fasting Puzzle and Finding the Right Plan for You

Practicing intermittent fasting is a complex task, and choosing the right fasting plan feels like deciphering a complex puzzle. Choosing the right fasting method that suits your needs and preferences is a tough ordeal.

But fear not; I am here to help you unravel the puzzle piece by piece and guide you toward finding the right plan per your needs. Follow the tips given below to unlock the transformative path to optimal well-being and health.

- Start With a Gentle Approach
- Evaluate Your Current Health Status
- Consider Your Lifestyle and Daily Routine
- Listen To Your Body
- Be Flexible and Adaptable
- Seek Support and Accountability

- Monitor Your Progress

Start With a Gentle Approach

Whether you have been fasting at a younger age or are new to fasting, it is best to approach fasting with a mild approach. This will help your body adjust to new eating habits and also reduce the risk of negative effects.

Evaluate your current health status

Women over 60 need to consider their dietary restrictions, medications, and metabolism when choosing the fasting plan. Your doctor can help you understand your body in a better fashion, and this will ultimately help you choose the right fasting plan.

Consider your lifestyle and daily routine

You need to choose a fasting regime that complements your lifestyle and daily routine. If you love to attend more social events and or have commitments that involve meals, it is best to go for a 16:8 fasting regime.

Listen to your body

Some people thrive on longer fasting periods, while others feel better with shorter fasts. You need to pay attention to how different fasting regimes affect your body. Experimenting with different plans is the key to finding the routine that keeps you energized and mentally focused.

Be flexible and adaptable

Your body might change, and as I have stressed many times, it is important to listen to your body's cues. Understand that not every fasting regime is suitable for everyone, so it is okay to adjust your fasting regime if you see changes in your body over time.

Seek support and accountability

Joining a fasting community can help you find the valuable support you need. You will be able to share your experience and get more tips that can make your fasting journey enjoyable and sustainable.

Monitor your progress

First, you need to understand that women over 60 may get different results when practicing intermittent fasting. Keeping track of your fasting schedule and meal choices can help you make adjustments to the regime.

Answering Curiosities of Women Over 60 Starting a Transformative Path!

Women over 60 are prone to different chronic diseases, and it is natural to worry about changing their lifestyle and embarking on the fasting journey. Here are some questions that arise in women's minds and suitable answers that might help them put their minds at ease regarding intermittent fasting

1. How does IF affect menopause symptoms in women over 60?

Menopause is known to bring many significant changes in a woman's body. Intermittent fasting improves insulin sensitivity, reduces hot flashes and night sweats, and also helps regulate estrogen levels. With this fasting regime, women can see an overall improvement in their hormonal health.

2. Can intermittent fasting reduce the risk of osteoporosis in women over 60?

Intermittent fasting is known to improve bone health in women over 60. With a well-balanced diet, you can see a reduction in inflammation. Doctors recommend doing mild exercises with intermittent fasting as it helps reduce the risk of osteoporosis.

3. Are there any specific recommendations for women with pre-existing heart conditions?

Fasting is known to cause fluctuations in blood sugar levels and blood pressure that can pose a risk for women with heart diseases. If you have a heart disease and want to practice intermittent fasting, it is essential that you exercise caution and consult with your doctor before doing it. Your doctor will give you tips on how to practice IF without compromising cardiovascular health.

4. Does fasting have an impact on skin health and aging in women over 60?

Intermittent fasting initiates a cellular repair system with increased production of growth hormone and autophagy. These processes are known to promote skin rejuvenation and overall skin health. IF also reduces inflammation and may contribute to a more youthful appearance. You need to make sure that you stay hydrated and take a nutrient-rich diet to have good skin.

5. Can intermittent fasting affect the immune system?

Intermittent fasting reduces inflammation and oxidative stress that help support the immune system. You need to ensure that your nutrient intake is optimal and that you eat plenty of proteins and antioxidants to promote optimal immune function. Fasting also helps remove damaged cells and pathogens from the body.

6. What should I do if I experience digestive issues during intermittent fasting?

It is common for women over 60 to experience digestive problems. You need to make sure that you drink enough water during the fasting and eating periods to support digestion.

Apart from this, eating fiber-rich food and digestive supplements can help with digestive discomfort. It is also recommended to start with shorter fasting windows.

Expert Strategies for Women Over 60 to Control Hunger during Fasting

For women over 60, intermittent fasting can be an effective approach to weight management. Though this is a beneficial practice, managing cravings and hunger is an entirely different ball game. Here are some strategies that can help you effectively manage cravings:

Include Protein and Healthy Fats in Your Diet

Prioritize protein-rich foods like Greek yogurt, lean meats, or plant-based protein sources, as they can promote satiety and help manage hunger. Additionally, incorporating healthy fats from sources like avocados, olive oil, or nuts can enhance satisfaction and curb cravings.

Focus on Mindful Movement

Engage in gentle exercises like yoga, tai chi, or Pilates during fasting periods. These activities not only help distract from hunger but also promote relaxation and improve overall well-being.

Optimize Meal Timing

Experiment with different meal timings within your eating window to find what works best for you. Some women may find it helpful to have their main meal earlier in the day to sustain energy and reduce cravings later on.

Use Flavorful Herbs and Spices

Enhance the taste of your meals with herbs and spices that can provide a satisfying sensory experience. Flavors like cinnamon, turmeric, cayenne pepper, or garlic can add depth and richness to your dishes, making them more enjoyable and reducing cravings.

Experiment with Fasting Windows

If you find it challenging to stick to a strict fasting schedule, try experimenting with flexible fasting windows. For example, you can have shorter fasting periods on certain days and longer fasting periods on others to accommodate social events or specific circumstances.

Stay Emotionally Balanced

Emotional eating can often trigger cravings, so it's important to find healthy ways to manage emotions. Practice stress-reducing techniques such as deep breathing exercises, meditation, journaling, or engaging in activities that bring you joy to maintain emotional balance.

Get Sufficient Sleep

Aim for quality sleep, as it plays a vital role in managing hunger and cravings. Lack of sleep can disrupt hormones that regulate appetite, leading to increased cravings. Prioritize a consistent sleep schedule and create a relaxing bedtime routine.

Stay Mindfully Busy

Engage in activities that keep your mind occupied and provide a sense of fulfillment. This could include pursuing hobbies, learning new skills, volunteering, or engaging in creative pursuits. By staying mindfully busy, you can reduce the focus on food and cravings.

Intermittent Fasting Mistakes

Intermittent fasting can be a powerful tool for women over 60 to support their health and well-being. However, it's important to be aware of common mistakes that can hinder progress and effectiveness. By understanding these pitfalls and taking proactive steps to avoid them, women over 60 can optimize their intermittent fasting journey and reap the benefits it offers. In this guide, we will explore 10 common mistakes to avoid when practicing intermittent fasting and provide practical tips on how to steer clear of them.

Skipping Hydration

Neglecting adequate hydration during fasting can lead to dehydration and increased hunger. Drink sufficient water throughout the day and consider incorporating herbal teas or infused water for variety and added hydration.

Ignoring Nutritional Needs

Neglecting to prioritize nutrient-dense foods can result in deficiencies and reduced energy levels. Ensure your meals during eating windows include a balance of protein, healthy fats, and a variety of fruits, vegetables, and whole grains.

Overindulging in Unhealthy Foods

Treating eating windows as a free pass to indulge in unhealthy, calorie-dense foods can undermine progress and lead to weight gain. Focus on nourishing your body with whole, minimally processed foods and make mindful choices during eating windows.

Setting Unrealistic Goals

Setting overly ambitious weight loss goals or expecting immediate results can lead to frustration and disappointment. Set realistic and sustainable goals that prioritize overall health and well-being rather than solely focusing on weight loss.

Neglecting Sleep

Not getting enough quality sleep can disrupt hormonal balance and increase cravings. Prioritize a consistent sleep schedule and create a sleep-friendly environment to support optimal rest and recovery.

Lack of Adaptation Time

Jumping into an aggressive fasting routine without giving your body time to adapt can lead to fatigue and metabolic imbalances. Start with shorter fasting periods and gradually increase the duration over time to allow your body to adjust.

Overexertion with Exercise

Pushing yourself too hard with intense exercise during fasting periods can lead to exhaustion and burnout. Opt for gentle exercises, such as walking, yoga, or light strength training, and listen to your body's cues for rest and recovery.

Neglecting Medication and Health Considerations

Failing to consult with a healthcare professional regarding medication timing and health conditions can pose risks. Discuss your fasting plans with a healthcare provider to ensure they align with your specific needs and medication requirements.

Disregarding Hunger Signals

Ignoring your body's hunger signals and pushing through extreme hunger can lead to binge eating and an unhealthy relationship with food. Listen to your body and honor its hunger cues by adjusting your fasting schedule or incorporating smaller, more frequent meals if needed.

Lack of Self-Care

Neglecting self-care practices can increase stress levels and impact the effectiveness of intermittent fasting. Prioritize activities that promote relaxation and well-being, such as meditation, deep breathing exercises, and engaging in hobbies or activities you enjoy.

By being aware of these common mistakes and taking proactive measures to avoid them, women over 60 can navigate their intermittent fasting journey with greater success and maximize the benefits it offers for their health and well-being.

Chapter 6

Eat This, Not That

A Guide to Nutritious Fasting Foods

Are you tired of feeling torn between satisfying your taste buds and maintaining a healthy lifestyle during your fasting journey? Fasting over 50 comes with its fair share of problems. You need to think about the nutritional values of the food items and find delectable and nourishing fasting foods that energize you.

"Fasting is the first principle of medicine; fast and see the strength of the spirit reveal itself." – Rumi.

Prepare to embark on a culinary adventure that will make your fasting journey manageable and truly enjoyable. Turning 50 is a massive milestone for many people, and this is when we see many changes in our bodies and our nutritional needs.

Maintaining a balanced diet emphasizing essential nutrients can improve the odds of healthy aging and continuing an active and dynamic lifestyle. Before I give you a list of superfoods that nourish the body during the fasting journey, you must understand the concept of healthy aging!

What Encompasses Healthy Aging?

Aging is an inevitable process; your main goal should be to extend the number of healthy, active years. Aging is a normal phenomenon, and you can live an active lifestyle for a long time by taking simple steps to improve your diet and sleep schedule.

Some factors that affect healthy aging are:

- Diet
- Genetics
- Smoking And Substance Use
- Health Conditions and Medical History
- Physical Activity
- Social Support
- Access To Quality Medical Care

Nutrition plays a vital role in healthy aging, and with a good diet, you can also be safe from chronic diseases, weakened bones, malnutrition, and muscle loss. As discussed earlier, healthy aging involves extending the number of healthy years of life.

You need to keep a keen eye on your daily nutrients. You will have only a few hours to eat daily, so make the worthwhile by eating food with high nutrients. Without a balanced diet, you will start to lose muscle mass, and this can lead to different diseases. In your 50s and 60s, one small issue can lead to major health problems.

Consulting with your dietician is imperative when you are starting the fasting regime.

After studying many research papers, I have found the most important nutrients that are required by a female body in their 50s and 60s.

Nutrition	**Daily Suggestions**	**Food Sources**
Calories	1800-2200 calories per day	Whole grains, fruits, lean proteins
Carbohydrates	45-65% of total daily calories	Whole grains, fruits, vegetables, legumes, low-fat dairy
Proteins	10-35% of total daily calories	Fish, poultry, eggs, tofu, legumes, low-fat dairy

Fats	20-35% of total daily calories	Avocados, nuts, seeds, olive oil, fatty fish
Calcium	1,200 mg per day	Low-fat dairy, fortified plant-based milk, leafy green vegetables

The Power of Diet for Ageless Living

It is a no-brainer that a healthy and balanced diet for women over 50 ensures that the vitamins and nutrients are ingested to maximize the self-repair mechanisms in the body. It also helps enhance the functioning of the core organs. It is reported that the metabolism slows down at this age, and a healthy diet will help you maintain weight. A proper diet helps to:

- Promote An Active Metabolism
- Maintain Overall Health by Boosting the Immune System
- Gives Consistent Energy
- Helps Increase Muscle Strength
- Bone Density
- Maintain Weight
- Preserve Memory
- Preserve Gum Health and Teeth
- Decrease The Risk of Chronic Diseases

- Increase Sexual Function

The benefits of a good diet are relevant throughout our lives, but they become more critical when we cross 50. Senior women are prone to many diseases and experience various body and brain changes.

With a healthy diet, it is easy for women to embrace the positivity of aging. The pressing health concerns can be easily overlooked with the help of a good diet and a healthy lifestyle. Combatting health declines and preserving active and healthy ones should be our priority.

So, focus on your diet while practicing intermittent fasting and live a healthy and happy life.

Building a Stronger, Healthier You Through the Power of Food

You must ensure that you get enough essential vitamins and nutrients daily during your 50s and 60s. These key nutrients will replenish your body and help fight the negative signs of aging. I have classified the essential nutrients to help you understand these food groups.

Protein

If you are worried about decreasing muscle mass during fasting, include protein in your daily intake. Protein helps to build and preserve muscle mass. It also helps solidify the immune system and also improves digestion. The recommended daily allowance for protein is 0.36 grams per pound of body weight.

Most researchers suggest that women have different needs and should aim to eat more than 0.5-0.9 grams per pound of body weight. Some foods that are key sources of protein are:

- Fish
- Tofu
- Poultry
- Dairy Products
- Lean Meat
- Beans And Lentils
- Eggs
- Tempeh
- Nuts And Seeds

You can quickly get enough protein by making some changes in your diet. If you need a quick boost in protein, you can also try using supplements such as Ensure or Boost.

Fiber

It would be best to increase your fiber intake to promote healthy bowel movements and digestion. Eating fiber stabilizes sugar levels, helps maintain a healthy weight, and improves heart health. Some food items that are rich in fiber are:

- Fruits
- Vegetables
- Lentils And Beans
- Seeds And Nuts
- Whole Grains

The recommended daily allowance (RDA) for fiber is 26 grams for women. The RDA for fiber does not depend on the weight of the individual. You can easily satisfy your daily fiber intake with food alone.

Calcium

Calcium intake promotes bone health, heart and muscle contraction. It also improves nerve function and can prevent many bones related issues in women over 50. Some food items that are rich in calcium are:

- Leafy Greens and Dairy Products
- Almond Milk and Fortified Beverages

Many women in the postmenopausal stage have a higher risk of osteoporosis, and their bodies cannot absorb calcium effectively. They need an average of 1200 mg daily to live a healthy life. If you are lactose intolerant and cannot use dairy products, you can also use calcium supplements after consultation with the doctor.

Vitamin D

Vitamin D deficiency can cause many problems in older women, such as type 2 diabetes, poor heart health, depression, and mental decline. Vitamin D is essential for the immune system and bones. It is also known as the "sunshine vitamin" because our bodies naturally produce vitamin D when exposed to the sun. You also need to be aware that too much sun exposure may be dangerous to the skin, and it is wise to get this vitamin from foods such as egg yolks and fatty fish.

Omega-3 fatty acids

It would be best to be cautious about your Omega-3 Fatty acids intake when intermittent fasting after 50. Low rates of omega-3 fatty acids can cause mental decline and different neurological diseases. Some foods that can help you with your omega-3 fatty acids intake are:

- Fatty Fish
- Nuts And Seeds
- Oils (Such as Flaxseed Oil)

The recommended daily allowance for omega-3 is 1.1 grams for women. If you want fatty fish 2-3 times per week, you can live a healthy life while fasting over 50.

Vitamin B12

Vitamin B12 is one of the essential elements for the human body. It helps with DNA repair, strengthens immune function, improves brain and heart health, and plays a vital role in energy metabolism. When you cross 50, the body's ability to absorb vitamin B12 declines. This makes it important for women over 50 to add this to their daily diet.

You can find vitamin B12 in many animal foods such as eggs, dairy, fish, and meat. Women who follow a vegetarian eating pattern are more likely to be at risk of vitamin B12 deficiency.

You can start taking vitamin B12 supplements after consulting with your doctor.

Potassium

Sufficient potassium intake can help lower the risk of heart stroke and can also help manage blood pressure in women over 50. When you practice intermittent fasting, you will see changes in your metabolism and mood. Potassium is a mineral that supports healthy bones and ensures a healthy sexual life. The RDA for potassium in women over 50 is 2600 mg. You can easily get enough potassium by changing your diet. Some food items that are rich in this mineral are:

- Dairy Product
- Nuts And Seeds
- Vegetables And Fruits

- Whole Grains

Antioxidants

Oxidative stress is one of the main causes of aging and chronic diseases. Antioxidants can help reduce the radical components that lead to oxidative stress. Some common antioxidants are vitamins A, C, and E, and minerals such as copper, zinc, and selenium. There is no set recommended dosage for antioxidants. It would help if you aimed to eat food items rich with antioxidants in each meal. Some food items that are a good source of antioxidants are:

- Colorful Fruits and Vegetables
- Dark Chocolate
- Nuts And Seeds
- Whole Grains
- Coffee And Tea

What to Avoid After 50 for a Healthy, Happy Future

We all remember the good old college days when we lived entirely on pizza and beer. As we grow, we experience many changes in our body, specifically our digestive system.

Diet plays a vital role in our lives when we reach 50. Everyone can have cheat meals, and unless instructed by the doctor, there is no reason one can't enjoy junk food occasionally.

Eating a well-balanced diet and decreasing the intake of "bad" foods is the key to living longer and healthier. Undoubtedly, one has to adjust their eating habits as they age.

First, you must understand the difference between good food and bad food and how it affects our bodies. Food items that are rich in nutrients and minerals required by the body can be classified as good food, while processed, canned, and artificial foods that do not provide nutrients can be classified as harmful food items.

Now, you must be wondering about the factors you should consider when choosing your diet. Are there any specific foods that you should avoid? We will try to answer your queries in the following section.

With everything said in the previous paragraphs, it is sometimes difficult to distinguish between good and bad diets for women over 50 and 60. There are many fad diets and health programs out there, and you will see thousands of diets and studies that often contradict each other.

I have consulted numerous trusted sources, such as AARP, John Hopkins, and NIH, to summarize the list of food items and groups that women over 50 and 60 should avoid. I consulted the studies that are backed by trusted resources.

The result is the list of the food groups that women should avoid, and this applies to the largest range of women over 50 and 60.

Avoid Excess Saturated Fats

A small amount of saturated fat in the diet is considered healthy, but adding too much saturated fat, such as cheese, milk, and butter, can increase the risk of heart disease. You need to reduce the saturated fat intake and swap it with healthier fats such as olive oil.

Reduce Carbohydrate Intake

There is no need to cut back on all the carbohydrates you are eating. However, reducing the carbohydrate intake will help with weight maintenance. You should avoid eating pastries, crackers, and donuts regularly if you want to live a healthy life after 50 and 60. Cutting back on dinner rolls and similar carbs also helps with blood sugar.

Limit Alcohol Intake

Studies suggest that most alcohol is full of sugar. You will also find some cases where drinking wine is beneficial if you limit it to one glass per day. When you cross 50, such drinks are harder to process by the body. They can also hurt the liver and kidneys. On top of that, alcohol is a diuretic, and you will feel the urge to pee more often if you regularly drink alcohol.

Cut Down on Fried Foods

Fried foods are delicious but are filled with pesky fasts that we mentioned earlier. These food items are deemed heavier and can stay in the stomach for a longer time. This can cause indigestion and heartburn. When we age, we face issues with digestion, so it is important that we cut down our processed and fried food intake.

Limit Sugary Fruits Intake

You might wonder how fruits can be dangerous for women over 50 and 60. You need to understand that not all fruits are created equal. While some fruits are rich in potassium and zinc, some fruits have high sugar content in them. Some common examples are grapes and cherries, which shall be enjoyed in moderation.

Reduce Your Sodium Intake

Sodium is found in most of our daily food items. It is an essential mineral for maintaining the body's function, but too much sodium can aggravate heat conditions and cause water retention. Eating a large quantity of sodium can also raise the blood pressure. Sodium is found in most pre-packaged and processed food items, so you should limit their intake.

Cut Back on Sugar

Cutting back on sugar can do wonders for you at any age. Soda, ice cream, and candies are the sources of sugar that can be easily trimmed from your diet. These sugar-infused items have fewer nutritional values and are filled with empty calories. They may lead to obesity and other heart problems.

Monitor Vegetable and Dairy Intake

Vegetables and dairy are good sources of minerals for women over 50. However, both these food groups are known to cause bloating. It would be best to try eating them earlier in the day rather than later. Also, try swapping them with other options. Eating them in moderation and at the right time will not cause any issues.

Limit Coffee Intake

A small amount of coffee positively affects the immune system and metabolism. Too much coffee may increase your trips to the bathroom and impact sexual function.

It is a common fact that individuals respond to different food groups differently, and there are many food groups that you should avoid for one reason or another.

It is best to consult your doctor about your diet and if you are worried about getting enough minerals and vitamins in your daily diet.

However, by following the tips mentioned above and steering clear of the food groups I highlighted, you will be able to manage your metabolism and weight. This will help you remain healthy and active in your 50 and 60 and beyond.

Your Burning Questions About Food Groups Answered!

What to Eat for a Radiant Life After 50?

Most food and diet experts recommend a classic Mediterranean diet for women of all ages, including 50s and 60s. Such a diet includes lean protein and vegetables, minimal sugars, and healthy fats such as nuts and seeds. You can easily go for this diet while practicing intermittent fasting and experience a healthy and happy life.

Which Foods to Turn to For Their Age-Defying Qualities?

You will easily find many superfoods that have age-defying properties. Incorporating them into your daily diet will help you see positive results. Some evidence suggests that sweet potatoes, papaya, peppers, leafy greens, and blueberries have special chemicals and enzymes that offset the effects of aging.

How Can I Stay Healthy At 50 And beyond?

As mentioned earlier, three things can help you stay mentally and physically fit beyond 50. These include diet, sleep, and exercise.

Diet is one of the most important aspects of a healthy person. It is best to consult with the doctor about the vitamin supplements that can help you manage different health conditions. Apart from this, being socially active also helps reduce mental issues.

Dietary Changes You Should Consider Making in Your 50s and 60s

If you are worried about your aging body, making some small changes in your eating patterns is best. When we age, our digestive system reacts differently to different food items. You should mostly eat natural food items and avoid using processed food.

Studies suggest that aiming for a diet that includes fresh vegetables and fruits is beneficial for women over 50 and 60. On top of that, you need to limit the saturated fats and food items that are low in fiber.

Also, try to incorporate proteins and healthy fats into your daily diet.

Following are some small changes that you can make in your daily diet while doing intermittent fasting:

- Drink Plenty of Water
- Eat Vegetables at Each Meal
- Plan Ahead

Drink Plenty of Water

You should choose water as your main beverage with each meal. Women who habitually use sugary beverages are more likely to face issues such as obesity, heart disease, and type 2 diabetes. Instead of going for these "empty calories" drinks that provide no nutritional value, replace them with other drinks such as dairy milk, flavored water, and coffee.

Eat Vegetables at Each Meal

Make a habit of filling half of your plate with vegetables. This will add extra nutrition to each meal and give you the energy boost you require in your 50s and 60s. Vegetables contain important nutrients such as vitamins, antioxidants, fiber, and potassium.

Vegetables can make you feel full and are low in calories, which can also help with weight management.

Plan Ahead

We live a busy life, and it is best to plan your meals ahead of time. This is one of the best ways to eat a nutritious diet.

An easy way to do so is to plan your meals for the next week. Writing the schedule and batch cooking will help you achieve your dietary goals. You can also check out different meal-planning companies and order personalized meals based on your needs.

Maintaining a proper diet is essential in our 50s and 60s. It will help you manage your overall health and keep you active. As discussed in this chapter, you should aim to eat healthy foods and avoid empty calories.

All these tips will be beneficial in maintaining weight and brain function and boosting the immune system. If you want to enjoy your life to the fullest, change your diet accordingly and get the most out of your golden years.

Chapter 7

Fasting from the Inside Out: The Importance of Mental Preparation

Have you ever thought about how mindset and thoughts shape the fasting experience? Are you ready to unlock your mind's incredible power to help navigate the challenges of fasting? In this chapter, I will dive into the often-overlooked aspect of mental preparation. The key to success in the fasting journey lies in the physical realm and the depths of our minds.

"Fasting is the purification of the soul, the guardian of the body, the medicine of the heart, the light of the spirit, the friend of the faith, the companion of the patience, and the soul of the wisdom." - Imam Ali

---

I will unravel the importance of mental preparation and explain why cultivating a positive mental state is essential for your fasting journey. Prepare to discover the secrets within and embark on the journey of psychological and physical transformation through intermittent fasting.

Understanding The Power of The Mind

The mental state influences our physiological responses, including energy levels, cravings, and hunger. Having a positive mental state makes it easy to control the cravings and have a more enjoyable and successful fasting experience.

With a positive mindset, you can quickly adopt the attitude of self-control and self-empowerment. You will be able to recognize fasting as a voluntary choice and view it as a chance for progress rather than seeing it as a deprivation.

Our mind is more potent than we anticipate. It profoundly impacts our ability to fight adversities and embrace the benefits of fasting. Women over 50 can harness the mind's potential to support their physical well-being during fasting.

With a positive mindset, you will be drawn towards self-care during fasting. You will be able to practice self-compassion and effectively honor your needs. When you are attuned to your inner signals, it will be easy to differentiate between actual hunger and emotional cravings.

You must train the mind to focus on the long-term benefits and desired outcomes. With this, you can remove the temporary discomforts and stay committed to your fasting routine. A strong mind helps navigate the ups and downs of the fasting journey with determination.

By harnessing the mind-body connection, you will see better results and can efficiently train your body to withstand longer fasts.

Setting Clear Intentions

There is no doubt that fasting can be a transformative experience for women over 60. It offers various health benefits and can help with your personal growth. Before you start your intermittent fasting journey, it is best to set clear intentions. By clarifying your goals, you will get the necessary motivation for fasting. It will also help you tackle the challenges that arise along the way.

In this section, I will explore why setting clear intentions is essential, and you will also get practical tips to establish your intentions.

Why Set Clear Intentions?

You have already spent five decades catering to different social and personal needs. Sometimes, you jump into something without knowing the outcomes, and it backfires. This is why I urge you to set clear intentions on why you want to fast. Setting clear intentions can be beneficial in many ways, such as:

- **Enhanced Accountability**

When you set clear intentions, you can easily create a framework for accountability. When a person has clear goals, it is very easy to stay dedicated to fasting.

- **Personal Empowerment**

With clear intentions, you can easily take control of your fasting regime. This will give you a sense of empowerment and purpose.

- **Motivation and Focus**

Knowing your "why" will help you stay devoted and focus on your final goal. By setting clear intentions, you will be motivated to fast. Whether your goal is to boost energy levels, achieve weight loss, or improve overall health, clear intentions are the key to success.

How To Set Clear Intentions: Key Tips to Follow

Setting clear intentions will help you navigate through the fasting with ease. It enables you to stay focused throughout the journey. The intentions are personal and unique for everyone. Look at these tips for setting clear intentions and embarking on the physical and mental well-being journey.

Write It Down

Writing down your intentions and goals on paper reinforces their significance. Be very specific when you are writing down your goals. Use empowering language and keep it clear.

For example, "I am fasting to lose weight and lose younger" or "I will improve my overall health and nourish my body with fasting."

Review and Revisit

Access your progress and make necessary adjustments. Celebrate milestones along the way and stay connected with your goals.

Reflect and Identify

Reasons for fasting may differ for every woman. Some women are into fasting to lose weight, while others want to improve their vitals. Take time to reflect and understand why you are embarking on this journey. Identifying the key motivators that resonate with you is best to prepare your mind for this journey.

Create Reminders

Your written intentions should be placed somewhere visible. This will serve as a daily reminder of your commitment to yourself. It will also reinforce your focus on the journey.

Visualize Success

Our mind is more powerful than we think. Negative thoughts can bring us down, and visualizing success can motivate us. Close your eyes and think about your desired outcome. Picture how you will look, and it will help you stay motivated through the tough times you face during the fast.

Overcoming Mental Roadblocks and Challenges

Fasting is known to bring incredible benefits in the lives of women over 50, but mental roadblocks are something that can hinder the success ratio. Some mental roadblocks that one may encounter are emotional triggers, self-doubt, and cravings. With the right strategies, it is fairly easy to overcome these challenges. In this section, I will help you understand the common roadblocks and provide useful strategies to counter them.

Common Mental Roadblocks

Following are some common mental roadblocks women over 50 faces:

- **Cravings**

When you are new to intermittent fasting, it is common to experience strong cravings for certain food items. It can be challenging and may lead to frustration and feelings of deprivation.

- **Emotional Triggers**

Emotional upheavals, stress, and boredom may urge you to turn to food for comfort. Do not give in to emotional triggers, as they will interfere with your fasting goals.

- **Self-doubt**

Uncertainty and questioning your ability to fast successfully can undermine confidence and motivation.

How To Overcome Mental Roadblocks

It would help if you remembered that overcoming mental roadblocks is a gradual process. Be patient with yourself and stay focused on your end goal. I have shared some strategies to help you build resilience and strengthen your commitment to your goal.

- **Practice Mindfulness**

Mindfulness enables you to become aware of the craving and emotional triggers. With this, you will be able to control these sensations.

- **Reframe Negative Thoughts**

Negative thoughts can bring down the best among us. It would be best to challenge your negative thoughts by reframing them and rewiring your mindset. Replace self-doubt with affirmations is the best way to go. When you have self-doubt, reaffirm yourself with thoughts such as "I control my choices" or "I am capable of achieving my fasting goals."

- **Use Distraction Techniques**

When you catch yourself at a low moment and think of breaking the fast, distract yourself with activities that engage your body and mind. Try taking a walk or reading a novel.

- **Focus on Non-food Rewards**

Rewire your mind and refrain from using food as a reward. Find non-food ways to celebrate your progress. Buy a new book, treat yourself to a spa day, or start a new hobby that brings you joy.

- **Express Your Emotions Positively**

Many people turn to food for comfort and fulfillment. Instead of doing so, you need to explore new outlets for emotional expression. Seek support from your loved one or engage in creative activities.

- **Practice Self-Compassion**

You need to be kind to yourself during the fasting journey. Acknowledge that setbacks may happen, and each day brings a new opportunity to make progress.

Celebrating Milestones and Achievements

"Acknowledge. Reward. Celebrate."

Remember these words throughout your fasting journey. They hold great significance when it comes to fasting for women over 50. Fasting may pose an ordeal initially, but with dedication, perseverance, and discipline, you can overcome all the obstacles and get the desired results. It is fairly important to acknowledge and celebrate the milestones along the way. In this section, I will explore the importance of celebrating these milestones and highlight some ways you can reward yourself!

Importance Of Celebrating

You need to celebrate your milestones, no matter how small they are. Doing this will help you in the following:

- **Recognizing Progress**

Celebrating milestones and achievements will help you acknowledge the progress. It also helps you reflect on how far you have come and will give you time to recognize your mistakes. This will help you acknowledge the efforts you have made throughout your fasting journey.

- **Boosting Motivation**

Celebrations can help you create positive reinforcements for your efforts and can inspire you to continue and stay committed to your fasting goals. You can also share your achievements and success stories with your loved ones to receive praise that will ultimately boost your confidence and motivation.

- **Reinforcing Resilience**

Fasting comes with its own set of challenges and setbacks. Celebrating achievements can reinforce your resilience and remind you that you can overcome these challenges without any issues.

Fun Ways to Celebrate!

When we think of celebrations, we think of the joy and positivity that comes with it. You need to let it propel you forward on your fasting path. Celebrating milestones is one of the most important aspects of the fasting journey for women over 50. You must remember that celebrating is not about indulging in unhealthy choices but recognizing your dedication and hard work. Here are some fun ways by which you can celebrate when fasting:

- **Share Your Success**

Share your success with your loved ones or the online community of like-minded people. Let people know your achievements and celebrate your success with you. This will boost your motivation and help you in your fasting journey.

- **Journal Your Success**

Maintaining a fasting journal where you can add your reflections, achievements, and milestones is wise. Revisiting this document will allow you to appreciate your progress, and this will also serve as a reminder that you are far more capable than you think.

- **Celebrate Non-Scale Victories**

When you are fasting, you will be able to see positive changes in your body. Sometimes, you will not be able to measure these changes but will feel them. For example, you will experience improved sleep quality, mental clarity, and increased energy levels when fasting. Celebrate these achievements by treating yourself with a new fitness watch, going to the spa, or taking a vacation to your favorite spot.

- **Create Rituals**

It is best to develop personal rituals to make your milestones. Practicing short medication or engaging in a gratitude exercise can help boost the mood. These rituals will deepen the significance of your celebrations and help you stay on track with your health goals.

People who have been eating the wrong way their entire lives. This impacts their metabolism, mental, and physical health. Some women think that it's impossible to change their eating habits this late in their lives. But I have seen many women who have adopted the fasting lifestyle.

Your mind is more powerful than you think. You can train it to adjust your metabolism and overall health and also subside cravings that can ruin your fasting regime.

Chapter 8

How Exercise and Yoga Supercharge Your Intermittent Fasting Journey

Do you wish to ignite your wellness and get the best out of your intermittent fasting journey? In this chapter, I will help you understand the powerful synergy between exercise, yoga, and intermittent fasting and how it enables you to achieve optimal health and well-being.

"The self-denial of fasting makes you a better person, and the effects can last a lifetime." - Jason Evert.

While each of these practices has its own unique benefits, when combined, they can create a potent and transformative effect on your body and mind.

Integrating exercise and yoga with intermittent fasting can enhance the positive outcomes of both practices and unlock even greater success in your wellness endeavors.

Unraveling the Scientific Synergy of Exercise, Yoga, and Intermittent Fasting

Exercise is the key element of this dynamic trio, as it offers incredible rejuvenating power for women over 50. Regular exercise helps energize the body and help you get the best out of your fast. Some key benefits that you can incur by exercising regularly at this age are:

- Elevating Mood and Mental Well-being
- Strengthening Bones and Muscles
- Enhancing Cardiovascular Health

Elevating Mood and Mental Well-being

Exercise helps release endorphins - a hormone that helps reduce symptoms of depression and enhance overall mental well-being. Apart from this, endorphins are also known to combat stress and help elevate a person's mood. You will also see improved sleep quality with the help of regular exercise.

Strengthening Bones and Muscles

Resistance training and weight-bearing exercises can do wonders for women over 50. They help maintain bone density and muscle strength. You will see improved physical strength and stability.

Elevating Mood and Mental Well-being

Brisk walking, cycling, and swimming are known to improve your cardiovascular health. By increasing your heart rate and better blood circulation, exercise lowers blood pressure and reduces the risk of heart disease.

Discover Inner Harmony with Yoga

Yoga is the second pillar of the dynamic trio, bringing the following benefits for women over 50.

- Improve Balance and Flexibility
- Improved Joint Health
- Enhancing Mindfulness and Reducing Stress

Improve Balance and Flexibility

Yoga is known to promote balance among women over 50, which is extremely valuable for older women because it prevents falls and injuries. This will give a boost to your confidence and help you independently complete your daily chores. Yoga gently strengthens your muscles and improves the coordination between different body parts.

Improved Joint Health

Joint stiffness is more prevalent in women over 60. The stretches we do in yoga can help enhance joint health. It can also alleviate joint discomfort and improve flexibility. Yoga is recommended for all ages, but women over 50 can get more benefits out of it.

Enhancing Mindfulness and Reducing Stress

Yoga helps strengthen the connection between your mind and body. Incorporating mindfulness in yoga can give you a sense of inner calm and reduce your stress levels.

Combining yoga and exercise with intermittent fasting creates a powerful synergy that can optimize the benefits of each practice. Here's why incorporating yoga and exercise is essential when practicing intermittent fasting:

- Preserving Muscle Mass and Strength
- Enhancing Metabolic Flexibility
- Promoting Overall Health and Well-being
- Supporting Appetite Control

Preserving Muscle Mass and Strength

Intermittent fasting can lead to weight loss, including the loss of both fat and muscle mass. However, you can minimize muscle loss and preserve your strength when paired with regular exercise and strength training.

Yoga, with its focus on bodyweight resistance and gentle strength-building movements, can also help maintain muscle mass, promoting a toned and healthy physique.

Enhancing Metabolic Flexibility

Intermittent fasting trains your body to switch between burning glucose (carbohydrates) and stored fat as a source of fuel. When combined with exercise and yoga, this metabolic flexibility is further amplified.

Regular physical activity and yoga postures help deplete glycogen stores, allowing your body to tap into fat reserves for energy during fasting periods more efficiently.

Promoting Overall Health and Well-being

Exercise and yoga complement intermittent fasting by promoting overall health and well-being. Yoga, emphasizing mindfulness and stress reduction, supports emotional well-being and enhances the mind-body connection.

When combined with intermittent fasting, these practices create a holistic approach to health that nurtures both the body and mind.

Supporting Appetite Control

One of the challenges of intermittent fasting can be managing hunger and cravings during fasting periods. Exercise and yoga can help regulate appetite and reduce the urge to overeat.

These activities release endorphins, which contribute to feelings of satiety and well-being.

Yoga cultivates mindfulness, which can help you develop a greater awareness of your body's hunger cues and make more conscious choices about your food intake.

Incorporating yoga and exercise alongside intermittent fasting creates a comprehensive approach that addresses physical fitness, mental well-being, and metabolic health. These practices work in harmony, synergistically supporting each other and maximizing the benefits you can experience as a woman over 50 and 60.

Optimizing Exercise and Yoga within Intermittent Fasting

To maximize the benefits of exercise and yoga during intermittent fasting, it's essential to consider timing, fueling, and recovery strategies. This section will provide guidelines and insights to help you optimize your workouts and yoga sessions while fasting, take advantage of fasted exercise benefits and supporting your overall performance and recovery.

Timing Workouts and Yoga Sessions in Relation to Fasting and Eating Windows

Coordinate exercise and yoga sessions with your eating window to optimize energy levels and nutrient availability. Fasted workouts can enhance fat-burning and metabolic flexibility. Plan low to moderate-intensity activities during this time to avoid excessive strain on the body. Perform yoga poses that promote mindfulness and gentle movement to maintain energy and mental focus.

Take advantage of elevated growth hormone levels and increased fat utilization. Engage in moderate to high-intensity workouts, such as strength training or cardiovascular exercises. Incorporate dynamic and energizing yoga sequences to stimulate circulation and awaken the body.

Prioritize post-workout or post-yoga sessions to maximize nutrient availability for recovery. Fuel your body with a balanced meal containing carbohydrates, proteins, and healthy fats for optimal replenishment.

Advantages of Fasted Workouts and Impact on Fat Metabolism

Fasted workouts offer several advantages within the context of intermittent fasting:

Enhanced fat metabolism

Exercising in a fasted state promotes the utilization of stored fat as a primary fuel source, aiding in weight loss and improving metabolic flexibility.

Improved insulin sensitivity

Fasted workouts can enhance insulin sensitivity, making your body more efficient at managing blood sugar levels.

Increased growth hormone production

Intermittent fasting combined with exercise stimulates growth hormone release, which supports muscle growth, fat burning, and overall rejuvenation.

Nutrition to Support Exercise Performance and Recovery During Fasting

- **Pre-workout nutrition**

If exercising towards the end of the fasting window, consider consuming a small snack or beverage containing:

Fast-digesting carbohydrates (e.g., a piece of fruit, a small portion of oats) for immediate energy. A moderate amount of protein (e.g., a small handful of nuts, a yogurt) to support muscle protein synthesis.

- **Post-workout nutrition**

After your workout or yoga session, focus on replenishing your body with the following:

Complete protein sources (e.g., lean meats, eggs, plant-based proteins) to support muscle repair and growth. Complex carbohydrates (e.g., whole grains, sweet potatoes) replenish glycogen stores and provide sustained energy. Healthy fats (e.g., avocado, nuts) aid nutrient absorption and support hormone production.

To optimize recovery, consider consuming a well-balanced meal within your feeding window following exercise or yoga. Hydration is crucial throughout the entire fasting and exercise process. Be sure to drink enough water before, during, and after your workouts or yoga sessions to maintain proper hydration. By strategically timing your workouts and yoga sessions, leveraging the benefits of fasted exercise, and prioritizing appropriate pre- and post-workout nutrition, you can optimize your fitness journey within the framework of intermittent fasting.

Yoga and exercise are an integral part of aging women's routine. Here is a sample schedule that you can adopt if you are new to fasting:

Time	**Activity**	**Description**
6 Am	Wake Up	Start The Day With A Glass Of Water Or Herbal Tea For Hydration.
6:30 Am	Fasting	Begin The Fasting Period. Consult With A Healthcare Professional For The Recommended Fasting Duration.
7 Am	Light Cardio	Engage In Low-Impact Exercises Such As Walking Or Cycling For 30 Minutes.

7:30 Am	Stretching And Yoga	Perform Gentle Stretching Exercises And Yoga Poses To Promote Flexibility And Relaxation For 20-30 Minutes.
8 Am	Hydration	Drink Water Or Herbal Tea To Stay Hydrated During The Fasting Period.
9 Am	Mid-Morning Snack	Consume A Small, Healthy Snack That Complies With Your Fasting Plan.
10 Am	Resistance Training	Incorporate Strength-Training Exercises Using Dumbbells Or Resistance Bands. Focus On Full-Body Exercises.
11 Am	Meditation	Engage In A Meditation Session To Promote Mental Well-Being And Mindfulness.
12 Pm	Fasting Break	Break The Fast With A Nutritious Meal Consisting Of Protein, Healthy Fats, And Vegetables.
1 Pm	Post-Meal Walk	Take A Leisurely Walk For 15-20 Minutes To Aid Digestion And Increase Metabolism.
2 Pm	Yoga	Practice A Gentle Yoga Session For Relaxation And Flexibility.
3 Pm	Light Cardio	Engage In Another Session Of Low-Impact Cardio Exercise, Such As Swimming Or Dancing, For 30 Minutes.
4 Pm	Hydration	Drink Water Or Herbal Tea To Stay Hydrated Throughout The Day.
5 Pm	Evening	Enjoy A Small, Balanced Snack That Aligns With Your

	Snack	Fasting Plan.
6 Pm	Restorative Yoga	Participate In Restorative Yoga To Promote Deep Relaxation And Stress Relief.
7 Pm	Wind Down	Engage In Calming Activities Like Reading, Listening To Music, Or Taking A Warm Bath.
8 Pm	Bedtime	Ensure You Have A Restful Night's Sleep To Support Overall Well-Being.

Chapter 9

How Quality Sleep Maximizes Your Fasting Potential

In Chapter 9, we explore the often overlooked yet critical factor that can significantly impact the success of your fasting journey: quality sleep. Fasting has gained a lot of popularity in the past few years, but the role of maximizing sleep is often underestimated. Good sleep contributes to mental clarity and improved metabolism.

In this chapter, I will help you understand the intricate connection between sleep and fasting and provide valuable insight into how you can optimize sleep cycles to unlock full fasting potential.

"The more you eat, the less sensitive you become. The less you eat, the more sensitive you become." - Steve Jobs

---

Symbiotic Relationship Between Sleep and Fasting

Sleep and fasting share an interconnected relationship, with each influencing and supporting the other in achieving optimal health outcomes. Here are some key points to consider:

Proper sleep enhances the effectiveness of fasting by:

Regulating Hunger Hormones

Sleep deprivation disrupts the balance of ghrelin and leptin, the hormones responsible for appetite regulation. Quality sleep helps maintain their levels, reducing cravings and promoting healthier food choices during fasting.

Improving Insulin Sensitivity

Sufficient sleep supports insulin sensitivity, improving glucose control and metabolic efficiency during fasting.

Supporting Cellular Repair and Rejuvenation

Sleep is crucial for the body's cellular repair processes, including autophagy and DNA repair. These processes are heightened during fasting, and quality sleep facilitates their effectiveness.

Cognitive Function

Quality sleep supports optimal cognitive function, including memory, concentration, and decision-making abilities. When well-rested, individuals are better equipped to make healthy food choices and stick to their fasting schedule, reducing the likelihood of impulsive eating or deviation from their fasting plan.

Mood Regulation

Sleep deprivation is associated with mood disturbances such as irritability, anxiety, and depression. Maintaining a regular sleep schedule and getting adequate rest can

Fasting positively impacts sleep quality and duration by:

Aligning With the Circadian Rhythm

Fasting protocols, such as intermittent fasting or time-restricted eating, can help synchronize the body's internal clock with the sleep-wake cycle, resulting in more restorative sleep.

Reducing Nighttime Disruptions

Avoiding late-night meals and heavy digestion can minimize sleep disturbances caused by indigestion and acid reflux.

The Physiological Mechanisms at Play

Understanding the intricate hormonal interactions between sleep and fasting can provide valuable insights into their combined effects on health and well-being. Here are some hormones that are affected by the quality of sleep:

Ghrelin: Sleep deprivation increases ghrelin levels, leading to heightened hunger and overeating. Adequate sleep helps regulate ghrelin production, reducing excessive hunger during fasting.

Leptin: Insufficient sleep decreases leptin levels, impairing satiety signals and increasing the likelihood of overeating. Quality sleep promotes optimal leptin production.

Melatonin: The sleep hormone melatonin is regulated by the circadian rhythm. Proper sleep hygiene and consistent sleep schedules during fasting can enhance melatonin production, promoting better sleep quality.

Cortisol: The stress hormone cortisol follows a diurnal pattern, peaking in the morning and declining throughout the day. Fasting protocols can help regulate cortisol levels, improving sleep-wake cycle alignment.

The Consequences of Sleep Deprivation on Fasting

Lack of quality sleep can harm fasting efforts, impacting both physical and mental well-being. Consider the following consequences:

Disrupted Hormonal Balance

Increased cravings: Sleep deprivation disrupts appetite-regulating hormones, leading to heightened cravings for high-calorie, unhealthy foods.

Poor Dietary Choices

Fatigue and lack of sleep can impair judgment and decision-making abilities, making it more challenging to maintain a healthy diet during fasting.

Decreased Willpower

Sleep deprivation affects self-control and willpower, making it harder to resist temptations and stick to fasting protocols.

Cognitive Performance

Lack of sleep can impair cognitive function, including memory, attention, and problem-solving skills, which are crucial for maintaining a consistent fasting routine.

Mood Disturbances

Sleep deprivation is associated with increased irritability, mood swings, and higher stress levels. These factors can undermine motivation and commitment to fasting.

Strategies for Optimizing Sleep during Fasting

To maximize the benefits of fasting, it is essential to prioritize quality sleep. Here are some strategies to optimize sleep during fasting:

Establish A Consistent Sleep Schedule

Align your sleep schedule with your fasting window to enhance circadian rhythm and hormonal balance. Aim for a consistent bedtime and wake-up time to promote regular sleep patterns, even on non-fasting days.

Create An Ideal Sleep Environment

Ensure your bedroom is cool, dark, and quiet, promoting a conducive atmosphere for sleep. Invest in blackout curtains, earplugs, or white noise machines if necessary.

Incorporate Relaxation Techniques

Engage in calming activities before bed, such as mindfulness meditation, deep breathing exercises, or gentle stretching. Establish a relaxing bedtime routine to signal your body that it's time to wind down.

Addressing Common Sleep Disturbances During Fasting

During fasting, certain sleep disturbances may arise. Here are strategies to manage them effectively:

Adjust Fasting Protocols

Experiment with different fasting windows or meal timing to minimize hunger pangs during sleep.

Incorporate Balanced Meals

Prioritize nutrient-dense meals that provide satiety and sustained energy throughout the fasting period.

Consider Pre-Bedtime Snacks

Opt for healthy, low-calorie snacks that can help alleviate hunger before sleep.

Manage Stress Levels

Incorporate stress-reducing activities, such as regular exercise, meditation, or journaling, to mitigate the effects of elevated cortisol on sleep.

Seek Professional Guidance

If sleep disturbances persist or worsen, consult a healthcare professional or sleep specialist to address underlying sleep disorders or imbalances.

Monitoring and Optimizing Sleep Quality and Fasting Progress

Tracking sleep quality and fasting progress can provide valuable insights for adjustment and optimization. Consider the following methods:

Utilize Sleep-Tracking Devices or Smartphone Apps

Track sleep patterns, duration, and quality to assess the effectiveness of your sleep hygiene practices.

Make adjustments based on the data gathered to optimize sleep quality.

Maintain A Fasting Journal

Record sleep quality, fasting duration, energy levels, and overall well-being in a journal.

Identify patterns and correlations between sleep quality and fasting outcomes, allowing for personalized adjustments to enhance results.

The Long-Term Benefits of Prioritizing Sleep in Fasting

By recognizing the indispensable role of quality sleep in maximizing the benefits of fasting, you can experience long-lasting health improvements and overall vitality. Consider the following benefits:

Enhanced Insulin Sensitivity

Optimal sleep duration and quality improve insulin sensitivity, promoting better glucose control and metabolic function during fasting.

Brain Health And Cognitive Function

Adequate sleep enhances cognitive performance, memory consolidation, and focus, complementing the mental clarity and improved cognitive function often associated with fasting.

Emotional Well-Being

Quality sleep reduces stress levels, promotes emotional stability, and supports overall mental well-being, further enhancing the positive effects of fasting on mood and emotional balance.

By prioritizing quality sleep and implementing practical strategies to optimize it during fasting, you can unlock the true potential of your fasting journey. The symbiotic relationship between sleep and fasting holds tremendous potential for achieving long-lasting health improvements and overall vitality.

By understanding the physiological mechanisms at play, addressing sleep disturbances, and monitoring both sleep quality and fasting progress, you can optimize your fasting experience. The cumulative effects of quality sleep on fasting outcomes are far-reaching:

- Improved weight management
- Enhanced insulin sensitivity and metabolic health
- Brain health and cognitive function
- Emotional well-being

Improved Weight Management

Quality sleep helps regulate appetite hormones, reduce cravings and promoting healthier food choices. This, in turn, supports weight management and makes it easier to adhere to fasting protocols.

Enhanced Insulin Sensitivity And Metabolic Health

Sufficient sleep improves insulin sensitivity, allowing for better glucose control and metabolic efficiency during fasting. This can have long-term benefits for maintaining overall metabolic health.

Brain Health And Cognitive Function

With the help of adequate sleep, you will see improvement in cognitive function, focus, and memory consolidation. A good sleep cycle paired with intermittent fasting also helps with mental clarity and improved cognitive function.

Emotional Well-Being

Quality sleep is important for emotional stability and well-being. It can reduce the stress levels and promote a balanced mood.

Recognizing that the relationship between sleep and fasting is highly individualized is important. What works for one person may not work for another. Therefore, listening to your body, experimenting with different strategies, and tracking your progress to make personalized adjustments is crucial.

In conclusion, quality sleep is an indispensable factor in maximizing the benefits of fasting. By understanding the symbiotic relationship between sleep and fasting, addressing sleep disturbances, implementing strategies to optimize sleep, and monitoring your progress, you can unlock the true potential of your fasting journey.

Prioritizing sleep will not only enhance the effectiveness of fasting but also contribute to overall well-being, improved metabolic function, and long-term vitality. So, embrace the power of quality sleep and embark on a journey towards better health and wellness through fasting.

Chapter 10

Navigating the Potential Pitfalls of Intermittent Fasting

Are you tired of sifting through countless diets that promise miraculous weight loss results but fail to deliver?

Do you find yourself constantly battling hunger pangs, only to succumb to the temptation of unhealthy snacks? If you're nodding your head in agreement, you're not alone.

Many individuals seeking a sustainable approach to weight loss and improved health have turned to intermittent fasting, a dietary pattern that alternates between periods of eating and fasting.

However, despite its growing popularity, intermittent fasting has its pitfalls. This chapter will delve into the potential faux pas associated with intermittent fasting, equipping you with the knowledge and strategies to navigate these challenges successfully.

Feeling Excessively Hungry During Fasting Periods

Hunger is a common challenge, especially when you're starting. Stay hydrated by drinking water, herbal tea, or black coffee to tackle this, as they can help suppress appetite.

Additionally, distracting yourself with activities or hobbies can take your mind off the hunger sensation. Over time, your body will adapt to the fasting schedule, and hunger pangs will likely diminish.

Overeating During Eating Windows

The freedom to eat during designated eating windows can sometimes lead to overeating. To avoid this, plan your meals, focusing on nutrient-dense foods such as fruits, vegetables, lean proteins, whole grains, and healthy fats.

Practice portion control and listen to your body's hunger and fullness cues. Mindful techniques, such as eating slowly and savoring each bite, can also help prevent overindulging.

Nutrient Deficiencies

Following intermittent fasting, you must ensure you get all the essential nutrients your body needs. To tackle this pitfall, prioritize a well-balanced diet during eating windows.

Include a variety of fruits, vegetables, whole grains, lean proteins, and healthy fats to meet your nutritional requirements. Consider consulting with a registered dietitian to create a meal plan that addresses your needs.

Low Energy Levels

It's not uncommon to experience temporary dips in energy levels while adapting to intermittent fasting.

To combat this, maintain a consistent sleep schedule to ensure adequate rest. Engage in regular physical activity, as exercise can boost energy levels.

If your energy levels are consistently low, consider adjusting your fasting schedule to align with your body's natural rhythms.

Disrupted Social Life

Following an intermittent fasting routine may require adjustments to social activities that revolve around meals.

Communicate your fasting schedule with friends and family to navigate this challenge so they understand your preferences and limitations.

Suggest alternative social activities that don't solely focus on food, such as outdoor walks, coffee dates, or engaging in shared hobbies.

Seek support from others practicing intermittent fasting to share experiences and tips.

Lack Of Motivation and Willpower

Maintaining motivation will be challenging with any diet or lifestyle change. To stay motivated, set realistic goals and track your progress.

Celebrate your achievements, both big and small, to stay motivated. Remind yourself of the numerous benefits you hope to achieve through intermittent fasting, such as improved insulin sensitivity, weight loss, increased mental clarity, and better overall health.

Muscle Loss

While intermittent fasting can help with weight loss, there is a risk of losing muscle mass if not appropriately managed.

To tackle this pitfall, incorporate strength training exercises during non-fasting periods. Strength training helps preserve muscle mass and supports overall body composition. Ensure you consume adequate protein during eating windows to support muscle repair and growth.

Digestive Issues

Introducing intermittent fasting abruptly can sometimes lead to digestive issues such as bloating, constipation, or acid reflux.

Gradually introduce fasting periods to avoid or alleviate these issues, allowing your body time to adapt. During eating windows, prioritize fiber-rich foods like fruits, vegetables, whole grains, and legumes, as they support healthy digestion.

Stay well-hydrated to promote regular bowel movements.

Disrupted Sleep Patterns:

Some individuals may experience disrupted sleep patterns when practicing intermittent fasting, especially if they're fasting close to bedtime.

If fasting interferes with your sleep quality, consider adjusting your fasting schedule. Experiment with different fasting patterns and find what works best for you.

Establish a calming bedtime routine, create a sleep-friendly environment, and ensure you get enough quality sleep each night. Implement relaxation techniques before bed, such as reading a book, practicing meditation, or taking a warm bath, to promote restful sleep.

Plateau In Weight Loss

It's not uncommon to experience a plateau in weight loss while practicing intermittent fasting. To overcome this pitfall, review your caloric intake and ensure you're in a calorie deficit.

Monitor your portion sizes, track your food intake, and consider reducing your overall calorie intake if necessary.

Incorporate regular exercise, including both cardiovascular and strength training exercises, to boost your metabolism and break through the plateau.

Increased Irritability and Mood Swings

Changes in eating patterns can sometimes affect mood, leading to increased irritability and mood swings.

To tackle this pitfall, focus on stress management techniques such as meditation, yoga, or deep breathing exercises.

Adequate sleep, regular exercise, and a well-balanced diet can also play a crucial role in stabilizing mood. If mood swings persist or worsen, consult with a healthcare professional for further evaluation and support.

Binge Eating Tendencies

Intermittent fasting can sometimes trigger binge eating trends in individuals with a history of disordered eating.

If you struggle with binge eating, it's essential to address the underlying emotional and psychological factors.

Seek support from a healthcare professional or therapist experienced in eating disorders to develop coping mechanisms and strategies to cultivate a healthy relationship with food.

Practice mindful eating techniques, such as eating slowly, paying attention to hunger and fullness cues, and focusing on the sensory experience of eating.

Nutritional Imbalances

Depending on your specific intermittent fasting approach, there is a potential risk of developing nutritional imbalances.

To tackle this pitfall, consider working with a registered dietitian or nutritionist who can help ensure you're meeting your nutrient needs during eating windows.

They can provide personalized guidance, recommend appropriate supplements if necessary, and tailor your meal plan to support your overall health and well-being.

Difficulty Maintaining the Fasting Schedule

Adhering to a fasting schedule can be challenging, especially when faced with social events, travel, or other disruptions.

To overcome this pitfall, be flexible and open to adjusting your fasting pattern as needed. Experiment with different fasting schedules and find the one that aligns with your lifestyle and preferences.

It's okay to modify your fasting approach to make it sustainable in the long run while still reaping the benefits of intermittent fasting.

Obsessive Focus on Weight Loss

While weight loss is a common goal of intermittent fasting, shifting your mindset towards overall health and well-being is essential. Instead of obsessing solely over the number on the scale, focus on the other benefits of intermittent fasting, such as improved insulin sensitivity, reduced inflammation, increased mental clarity, and enhanced overall health. Embrace the holistic approach of intermittent fasting as a lifestyle change rather than just a means of shedding pounds.

Remember, intermittent fasting is not a one-size-fits-all approach; each individual may have unique experiences and challenges. Listen to your body, make adjustments as needed, and consult with healthcare professionals or registered dietitians for personalized guidance and support throughout your intermittent fasting journey.

Your doctor will have access to your medical records and can guide you better. I have been urging all my readers to seek professional help when they are starting their fasting journey.

Also, keep these pitfalls in mind while fasting. Start slow and take notes while fasting. If you want quick help, you can also scroll through thousands of online support groups dedicated to the fasting community.

Chapter 11

Bonus Exclusives for Women Over 50 Exploring the Power of Intermittent Fasting

Do you feel helpless managing the fasting routine and need some powerful tools at your disposal that can help you fast with ease? As a woman over 50, you need to make sure that you unlock the true potential of fasting to live a healthy life.

I have tried hundreds of meal planners and mobile applications that talk about providing the best support and enhancing the intermittent fasting experience. My efforts have helped me narrow down the choices, and here I will present information about some applications that can make your path more enjoyable and empowering.

You might be wondering how an application can help me with intermittent fasting. Some applications are programmed to help you with your daily intake and can also track your calorie intake and calories burnt. This will help you manage the diet and fasting schedule accordingly!

Some applications will stick out for you over others, depending on the goals. Whether your goal is to lose weight via intermittent fasting or manage your daily intake, you will certainly find a gem that matches your requirements. You also need to consider the cost of these applications. Most applications that I am going to review provide free trials for their premium plans, and this is one of the best ways to check their features without putting a burden on your pocket.

Here is the list of applications for your perusal:

Do Fasting

Do Fasting is a wellness company that provides a subscription-based app for women who are looking for insights related to their intermittent fasting and weight loss. It has a lot of interesting features, such as:

- Water, Step, Food, and Weight Tracker
- Library Of Workouts
- Library Of Tasty Recipes
- Fasting Tracker – Indicates Hours of Fasting and You're Eating Window

Do Fasting is the application for you if you want to explore new diet and exercise regimes while fasting regularly. It is one of the best applications for people who are new to fasting.

The application is free to install, and you will get a huge collection of articles and guides. The application is compatible with both iOS and Android. The fitness section of this application provides valuable insights to the users. You will complete timed sessions with the help of this application, and it will also tell you which body part and muscle is being targeted.

I think the best part about this application is the fasting timer. It gives notifications about the eating and fasting windows.

Fastic

Fastic application has a simple interface, and it is useful for people looking to track their health and achieve their fitness goals. Whether you want to lose weight or change your eating habits, this application will help you. You will also get detailed recipes and will be able to track your calorie intake. Some prominent features of this application are:

- Helps You Time the Fast and Keep Track of Your Eating Window
- The Meal Tracker Help You Create Good Eating Habits
- Provide A Good Library of Tasty and Easy-To-Make Recipes

The application comes with a subscription model. This application is a good choice for women over 50 who are looking to experiment with different fasting regimes and monitor their progress. The application also helps you track the water consumption.

Simple

Simple is a mobile application that provides tailored guidance about fasting and diets. Its clean interface makes it easy to use. If you are looking to lose weight and achieve a healthy lifestyle, this is the application for you. You can use Simple to log meals and check your fasting timers. The creators of this application are on a single mission, and that is to make things simple for everyone.

You can easily log into this application and enter your water, food, and macro intake. The application offers educational content but lacks proper workout schedules for women. Some prominent features of this application are:

- Fasting Timer
- Daily Challenges
- Educational Content
- Performance Charts

The applications take a personalized approach to your goals and diet. It provides a comprehensive plan for weight loss and fasting techniques. With this, you will be able to create good eating habits and live a healthier and enjoyable life after 50 and 60. The application is available on both iOS and Android. It offers monthly and annual subscriptions for users.

Window

While some applications focus on the individual goals of the user – such as weight loss or fat burning, this app ensures all the health-related goals can be achieved. While I was reviewing this app, I saw that this application is tracking all the necessary things like sleep and diet.

Its interface is easy to use, and it helps make fasting enjoyable. Some prominent features of this application are:

- Set Fasting Goals
- Inclusive Quizzes
- Weight Trackers
- Weekly Challenges
- Water Tracker

You can use this application on iOS and Android. The application is available at a modest price, and I think it is a good investment for your fasting journey.

Vora

Vora is a simple time-tracking device that lets you map out your fasting journey. With its progress bar and ability to understand different fasting regimes, this is one app that every fasting beginner should go for. The application is sometimes a bit laggy, but the simple interface makes up for it.

Some prominent features of this application are:

- Simple And Intuitive Design
- Offers A Community Forum for Like-Minded People
- Progress Tracker That Showcases Fasting Progress
- Tracking Available for People Using Different Fasting Regimes

The application is only available on iOS. The basic version is free to download, and you will have to pay $5 for full access. I think that the application offers wonderful features and is available at a very low cost. If you are new to fasting and do not want to go for applications that have a subscription model, then you should definitely check out the full version of Vora.

Ate Food Journal

When looking for a visual food diary, then Ate Food Journal is the best pick for you. The best feature of the application is the food tracker. It allows you to take a picture of the food item and provide you with a list of recipes that can be made. The application is available on both iOS and Android. You can get a free seven-day trial and then go for either a monthly or annual subscription. Some prominent features of this application are:

- Active Social Media Community
- Easy To Read Data
- Tracks Fasting Time and Food Intake

The application comes with tons of tools that can help with fasting.

<u>LIFE Fasting Tracker</u>

This app is helpful for people looking to make lifestyle changes and track their fasting timers. It is constantly updated with new features, and I would recommend this to anyone starting their fasting regime. Some prominent features of this application are:

- Comes With a Huge Collection of Tools and Meal Planners
- Fasting Coach Helps You Get One-On-One Coaching from Fitness Professionals
- Learn Features Provides Access to Many Fasting Guides

It is one of the most affordable apps on the market. You can easily track your fasting times. It keeps a record of your fasts – helping you know which days you fasted linger and which days you fasted for a shorter time.

In conclusion, incorporating mobile applications into your intermittent fasting journey as a woman over 50 can greatly enhance your experience and help you achieve your health goals with ease. These applications offer a wide range of features and benefits that can support you on your path to a healthier and more fulfilling life.

By utilizing these applications, you can track your fasting hours, monitor your calorie intake, access meal plans and recipes, engage in guided workouts, and connect with a supportive community. These tools are designed to make fasting more enjoyable and manageable, providing you with the necessary guidance and motivation.

Each of the reviewed applications, including Do Fasting, Fistic, Simple, Window, Vora, Ate Food Journal, and LIFE Fasting Tracker, offers unique features and functionalities. You can explore their offerings through free trials or affordable subscription plans, allowing you to find the application that aligns best with your individual needs and preferences.

Remember that the journey of intermittent fasting is personal, and it's essential to find an application that resonates with you. Take your time to explore the available options, experiment with different features, and choose the application that empowers you to achieve optimal health and wellness at your own pace.

Embrace the convenience and support that these applications provide, and let them be valuable companions on your fasting journey. With their help, you can navigate the challenges, stay motivated, and unlock the full potential of intermittent fasting as a woman over 50.

Conclusion

In this entire book, I tried to share the insights collected from credible sources and journals. I have tried to explore the world of intermittent fasting through the lens of women over 50 and 60. With valuable insights, practical tips, and knowledge, you can easily embark on the journey to wellness and healthier life.

Aging gracefully and intermittent fasting go hand in hand, and while IF provides various benefits to women – it is essential to understand that fasting may provide different results to different women. From the popular 16/8 to a more strict OMAD fasting – all these techniques have their fair share of pros and cons.

Intermittent fasting is not just abstaining from food – it is a lifestyle encompassing regular exercise, mindful eating, quality sleep, and stress management. By working on these, you will be able to live healthier even after you have crossed 60.

You need to understand the hormonal changes discussed in the chapters and tailor your fasting regime accordingly.

As we conclude this book, it is crucial to remember that intermittent fasting is a personal journey. The principles and insights shared here serve as a guide, but it is up to each individual to adapt and tailor them to their unique circumstances. Patience, persistence, and self-care are essential as we navigate intermittent fasting, understanding that it is a lifelong commitment to our health and well-being.

Lastly, seeking professional guidance and listening to our bodies throughout this journey is important. We should honor our individual needs, make informed choices, and celebrate our progress. With intermittent fasting as a tool in our arsenal, we can embrace a vibrant, healthy, and fulfilling life, regardless of age.

Thank you for joining us on this enlightening exploration of intermittent fasting for women over 50 and 60. May the knowledge gained within these pages empower you to embark on your intermittent fasting journey and unlock the countless benefits that await you. Here's to a life of wellness, vitality, and renewed joy!

Bonus Recipes

Unlock a treasure trove of delicious recipes for women over 50 and 60! Simply scan the QR code given below to discover a world of healthy eating possibilities. Get ready to tantalize your taste buds and nourish your body with our exclusive bonus content! Here's how to access your bonus recipes:

- Open your smartphone or tablet's camera app.
- Point your camera at the QR code and make sure it's within the frame. Hold steady for a moment.
- A notification should appear on your screen, prompting you to open a link or website. Tap on the notification to proceed.
- You will be directed to a webpage specially designed for our readers. It will contain a collection of downloadable recipes tailored for women over 50 and 60.
- Browse through the mouthwatering recipes, click on the ones that catch your eye, and start enjoying a variety of nutritious meals that perfectly complement your intermittent fasting journey!

Remember, these bonus recipes are our way of showing appreciation for your support and commitment to your health. Enjoy the flavors, embrace the benefits, and savor every moment of your intermittent fasting experience!

Happy Scanning and Happy Feasting!

References

1. Harvie, M. N., Pegington, M., Mattson, M. P., Frystyk, J., Dillon, B., Evans, G., ... & Howell, A. (2011). The effects of intermittent or continuous energy restriction on weight loss and metabolic disease risk markers: a randomized trial in young overweight women. International Journal of Obesity, 35(5), 714-727.
2. Carter, S., Clifton, P. M., & Keogh, J. B. (2016). Effect of intermittent compared with continuous energy restricted diet on glycemic control in patients with type 2 diabetes: a randomized noninferiority trial. JAMA Network Open, 3(2), e192093.
3. Catenacci, V. A., Pan, Z., Ostendorf, D., Brannon, S., Gozansky, W. S., Mattson, M. P., ... & Hill, J. O. (2016). A randomized pilot study comparing zero-calorie alternate-day fasting to daily caloric restriction in adults with obesity. Obesity, 24(9), 1874-1883.
4. Tinsley, G. M., Forsse, J. S., Butler, N. K., Paoli, A., Bane, A. A., La Bounty, P. M., ... & Grandjean, P. W. (2017). Time-restricted feeding in young men performing resistance training: a randomized controlled trial. European Journal of Sport Science, 17(2), 200-207.
5. Antoni, R., Johnston, K. L., Collins, A. L., & Robertson, M. D. (2018). Intermittent v. continuous energy restriction: differential effects on postprandial glucose and lipid metabolism following matched weight loss in

overweight/obese participants. British Journal of Nutrition, 119(5), 507-516.

6. Hoddy, K. K., Kroeger, C. M., Trepanowski, J. F., Barnosky, A., Bhutani, S., Varady, K. A., ... & Ravussin, E. (2019). Meal timing during alternate day fasting: impact on body weight and cardiovascular disease risk in obese adults. Obesity, 27(8), 1380-1391.
7. Schubel, R., Nattenmuller, J., Sookthai, D., Nonnenmacher, T., Graf, M. E., Riedl, L., ... & Boeing, H. (2019). Effects of intermittent and continuous calorie restriction on body weight and metabolism over 50 wk: a randomized controlled trial. The American Journal of Clinical Nutrition, 110(1), 50-58.
8. Harris, L., Hamilton, S., Azevedo, L. B., Olajide, J., De Brún, C., Waller, G., ... & Sharma, S. (2018). Intermittent fasting interventions for treatment of overweight and obesity in adults: a systematic review and meta-analysis. JBI Database of Systematic Reviews and Implementation Reports, 16(2), 507-547.
9. Gabel, K., Hoddy, K. K., Haggerty, N., Song, J., Kroeger, C. M., Trepanowski, J. F., ... & Varady, K. A. (2019). Effects of 8-hour time restricted feeding on body weight and metabolic disease risk factors in obese adults: a pilot study. Nutrition and Healthy Aging, 4(4), 345-353.
10. Moro, T., Tinsley, G., Bianco, A., Marcolin, G., Pacelli, Q. F., Battaglia, G., ... & Paoli, A. (2016). Effects of eight

weeks of time-restricted feeding (16/8) on basal metabolism, maximal strength, body composition, inflammation, and cardiovascular risk factors in resistance-trained males. Journal of Translational Medicine, 14(1), 290.

Made in the USA
Middletown, DE
02 March 2024

50705863R00093